The Beginner's Guide to
GROWING CANNABIS
and Making Your Own Healing Remedies

Tammi Sweet, MS

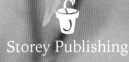

Storey Publishing

MY DEEP GRATITUDE and indebtedness to the green being, cannabis; thank you for all the ways you've helped me be a better human. Thank you to all the generous and loving growers of this beautiful plant who have shared their hard-won wisdom of how to work with her. This book would not be possible without you.

The mission of Storey Publishing is to serve our customers by publishing practical information that encourages personal independence in harmony with the environment.

Edited by Liz Bevilacqua
Art direction by Ian O'Neill
Book design by Ash Austin and Ian O'Neill
Text production by Liseann Karandisecky

Cover photography by © Tammi Sweet, except © Jose Coello/Stocksy, front (b.m.); Kris Miller/courtesy of the author, back (author); Mars Vilaubi © Storey Publishing, LLC, back (t.r.); © viennetta/Shutterstock.com, front (b.l.); © VISUALSPECTRUM/Stocksy, front (b.r.)
Interior photography by © Tammi Sweet
Additional photography by © Eddie Pearson/Stocksy, 114–116; Enecta Cannabis extracts/Unsplash, 129 l.; Kris Miller/courtesy of the author, iv, 80; Mars Vilaubi © Storey Publishing, LLC, i, iii, 18 l., 19–21, 40–41, 51, 54–56, 58–59, 61, 66, 74–76, 77 t., 86, 88–89, 96–99, 102–108, 129 r.; Pat Floyd/courtesy of the author, 52, 124; © Shawn Sweet, 69; Suzanne Johnson/courtesy of the author, 133 t.

Text © 2023 by Tammi Sweet

This publication is intended to provide educational information on the covered subject. It is not intended to take the place of personalized medical counseling, diagnosis, or treatment from a trained health professional. Know and obey any cannabis-related laws that may apply to you and your location. Please exercise caution when using health remedies of any kind and follow all safety guidelines.

Storey books are available at special discounts when purchased in bulk for premiums and sales promotions as well as for fund-raising or educational use. Special editions or book excerpts can also be created to specification. For details, please send an email to special.markets@hbgusa.com.

Storey Publishing
210 MASS MoCA Way
North Adams, MA 01247
storey.com

Storey Publishing, LLC is an imprint of Workman Publishing Co., Inc., a subsidiary of Hachette Book Group, Inc., 1290 Avenue of the Americas, New York, NY 10104

ISBNs: 978-1-63586-558-5 (paperback); 978-1-63586-559-2 (ebook)

Printed in Canada by Transcontinental Printing
10 9 8 7 6 5 4 3 2 1

Library of Congress Cataloging-in-Publication Data on file

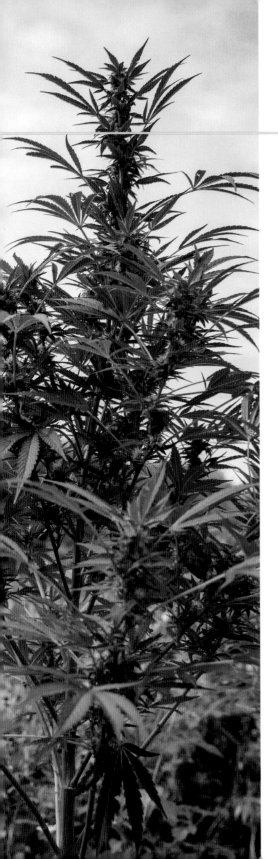

Contents

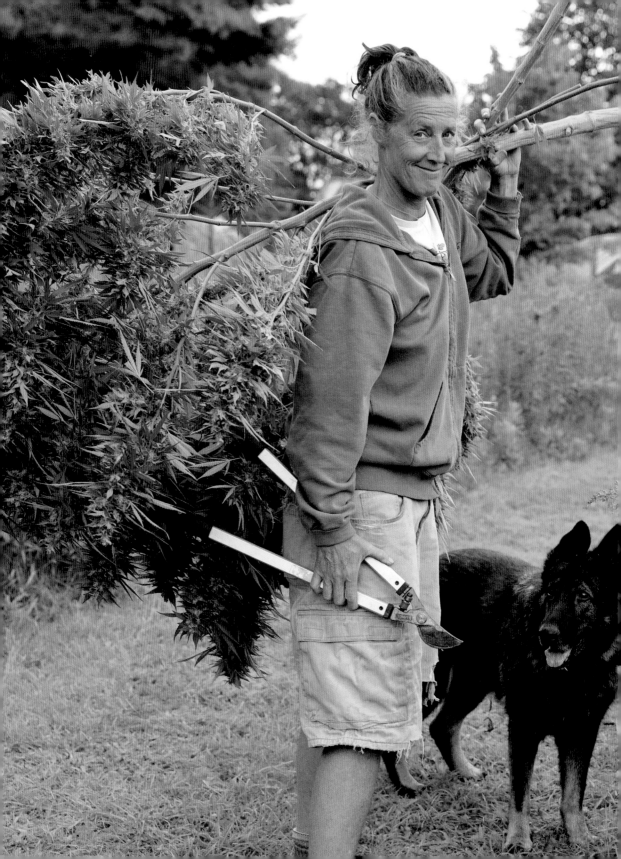

Welcome to the World of Growing Cannabis

Cannabis is a remarkable plant with the capacity to support healing and alleviate suffering. The plant is high in vitamins A, C, E, and beta-carotene; rich in protein, carbohydrates, minerals, and fiber; and has an ideal ratio of omega-6 to omega-3 fatty acids. Cannabis is also adaptive and gentle; it can ease anxiety, help with sleep, and provide relief from pain. It's no wonder cannabis has been used for health and healing for at least 6,000 years.

Perhaps you've been using CBD products purchased from a dispensary or other store and experienced some of the beneficial effects of cannabis. Perhaps you're a gardener who wants to grow a few cannabis plants yourself. Maybe you are curious about creating your own home remedies—salves, tinctures, oils, and more—to benefit from the healing properties of this plant.

Well, when it comes to healing, people experience a difference between industrially produced medicine and conscientiously cultivated medicine. The environment that cannabis plants are grown in, the nutrients used, the soil, and how the grower interacts with the plant are all important factors to consider when using medicine.

The best way to know what's in your cannabis remedies—and to understand how to craft medicine for your specific body and the specific outcomes you want—is to grow your own plants and make your own medicine. This way, you will know exactly where the flowers come from, how they are grown, and how the medicine is made. Growing cannabis yourself and making remedies from your plants will result in medicine that is better for you, more potent, and more targeted to your unique physiology.

As an herbalist, my goal is to help people gain greater knowledge of and respect for the cannabis plant and its healing properties, and to empower people to have the confidence to work with the plant.

Western medical practice would have us believe that we can separate the body into parts, isolate certain structures, understand their functions, and then prescribe how to fix them. In my experience, this does not work when dealing with a complex, living human being. Nothing in our bodies works in isolation. Herbalists understand that when you are dealing with a plant with thousands of active constituents, you simply cannot measure the effects of any individual constituent. Further, what happens inside one human body will not be exactly the same in the next person. I have a holistic approach to healing the body, growing plants, and making medicine.

When you buy cannabis products from a store, big company, or dispensary, you don't know what process the manufacturer has gone through to create the product. Some producers put the entire plant through a wood chipper, isolate one cannabinoid, process it into a white powder, and sell it as isolate or distillate. If they are using industrial heaters to quickly dry the plant material, most of the important medicinal elements are lost. Unless you ask specific questions, you won't know what is or isn't in the product you are buying and hoping to use for medicine.

Cannabis you grow yourself is far superior to large-batch industrial-grown

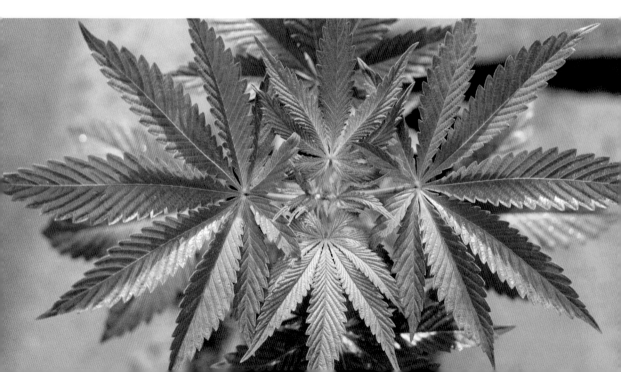

and -made medicine because you know everything that went into the growing of the plants, including your time, energy, and intentions.

For herbalists, whole-plant medicine means using all the parts of a plant containing the constituents needed for healing. In the case of cannabis, the medicinal parts are any part of the plant containing the crystally jewels—the trichomes. Most of the trichomes are found on the female flowers and the small leaves within and around the flowers. Basically, the trichomes are anything that sparkles.

We don't make our medicine by extracting only specific components to create chemical cocktails. When using all of the parts of the plant, containing all of the constituents, we benefit from all of the phytochemicals working together, including the fats, chlorophyll, and all of the cannabinoids in the trichomes. We humbly recognize that we don't know everything that's going on in the synergistic symphony of chemicals within medicinal plants, cannabis included.

In whole-plant medicine, we use all the constituents contained within the trichomes of the flower. Scientific studies on the effectiveness of cannabis medicine have overwhelmingly shown that whole-plant extracts are more effective than the separate constituents found in cannabis isolate or distillate. Whole-plant extracts are up to 330 times more effective, depending on the study. This proves what herbalists have always known about the synergistic, organic benefits of whole-plant medicine.

The holistic approach to healing requires looking at the whole picture, including the person seeking treatment, the health condition being addressed, the cultivar of the plant used for medicine, its growing environment, and the dosage. Every part of the equation is important and contributes to healing.

The deep and profound connection between humans and cannabis is the foundation for our healing with this amazing plant. The more we interact with her and the more we understand how our internal chemistry interacts with hers, the greater potential we have for healing ourselves naturally with all the gifts she has to offer.

Tammi

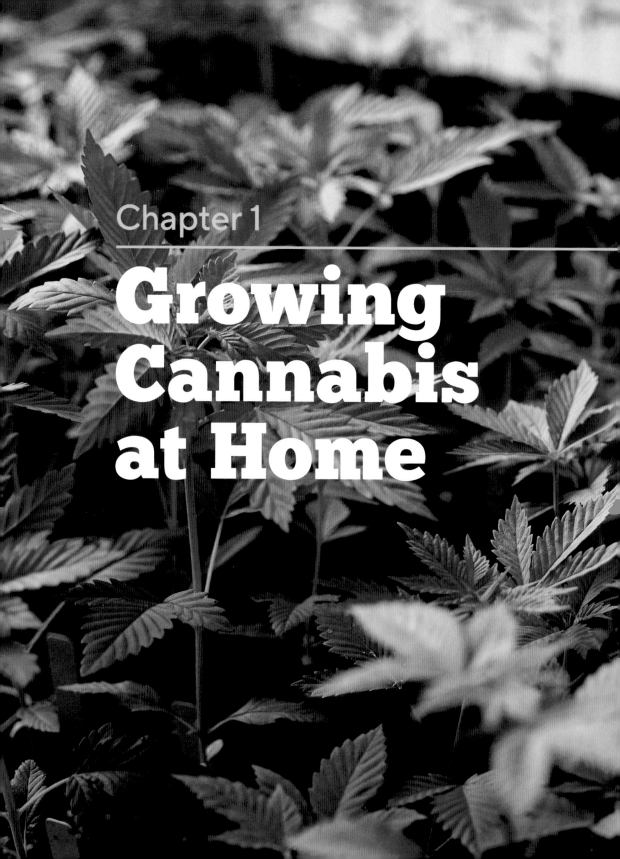

Chapter 1

Growing Cannabis at Home

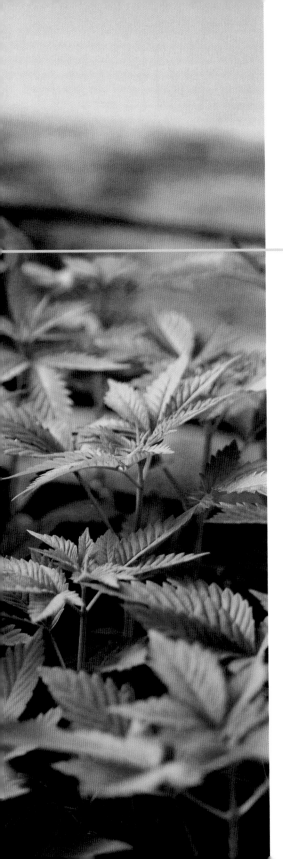

Cannabis grows as an annual plant, completing its life cycle in less than a year. A seed planted in spring will grow through summer into a tall plant that will flower in late summer through fall. If it has been fertilized, the plant will produce seeds to complete its life cycle, and its seeds will start the cycle again the following spring.

An Overview of the Process

Depending on where you live and what space you have available, you can start growing cannabis seedlings indoors and then move them outdoors or you can start them outdoors and keep them there. You'll start seeds in standard seed-starter pots like you'd use to grow tomatoes. You may have to move the plants to bigger pots if they outgrow the nutrients in the smaller pots. Then you will plant them into the ground. You can also transplant them into big containers if you prefer. To get the largest plants, well-nourished and well-drained soil in the ground is your best bet. If you decide to plant in pots, go big or go home.

Where I live in the Northeast (USDA Plant Hardiness Zone 5), I start my seedlings in April. I bring them outside into a protected spot in May and transplant my plants outside into garden beds in the first week of June. The first major pruning begins in mid-July. Flowering occurs mid- to late August. Flowers grow for 8 to 10 weeks, and harvest happens from late September into October depending on the variety and finish time.

Cannabis by All Names

The cannabis industry calls plants that are high in THC marijuana, weed, pot, or recreational. Because the word *marijuana* has been used to associate negative attributes with the plant and the brown peoples who worked with the plant, I don't use this nomenclature. I don't like using the word *hemp* either because it tries to distance high-CBD cannabis cultivars from high-THC ones. There is a movement to try to characterize CBD as the "good" constituent and THC as the "bad" constituent; but neither is good nor bad; they just have different properties. I use the term *cannabis* for both high-CBD and high-THC cultivars, because it is *all cannabis*.

Choosing a Cultivar

A cultivar is a variety of cannabis that has been cultivated through selective breeding. "Cultivar" is another term for variety or strain. There are hundreds of cultivars, with names like Bubba Kush, Pineapple Express, Blueberry Muffin, Diesel, Purple Haze, and many more. All the varieties you hear about or see at dispensaries are descendants from an original lineage and are either *Cannabis indica indica* or *Cannabis indica afghanica*. They are subtle variations within a subspecies that contain different terpene profiles and cannabinoid content.

SATIVA AND INDICA

If you step into a dispensary or talk with a grower, you will inevitably be asked if you are looking for "indica" or "sativa." This is how the industry talks about cannabis.

Cannabis is classified by the plant's leaf shape as well as the levels of CBD and THC present in the plant. Briefly, CBD is the chemical constituent in the plant that has a soothing effect on the body, is anti-inflammatory, and stimulates our own endocannabinoid system. Plants high in CBD and low in THC are commonly called hemp. THC is the constituent that regulates pain, is anti-inflammatory, and makes those who take it feel "high," among other things. In the realm of THC-dominant cultivars, people refer to tall, lanky plants that are energizing and heady as *sativa*, and they call short, squat plants that are sedating *indica*. For the record, you cannot determine a plant's sedative or energizing properties, or whether it is high in CBD or THC, simply by looking at it.

It is less important to find the particular "flavor of the month" cultivar of cannabis and more important to know what effects you are looking for—sedating or energizing

Chemical Constituents

THC (TETRAHYDROCANNABINOL) is the chemical constituent in the cannabis plant that is typically euphoric. It regulates pain, is anti-inflammatory, and gives people the "high" feeling.

CBD (CANNABIDIOL) is the chemical constituent in the cannabis plant that has a soothing effect on the body. It is also anti-inflammatory, and it gives people a feeling of relaxation.

TERPENES are chemical compounds in the cannabis plant that give the plant its distinctive smell. They are highly medicinal essential oils.

or calming—and then grow a cultivar that matches what you are looking for. The name of the cultivar means nothing when compared to the effect you are seeking. Reputable seed suppliers will be able to direct you to an appropriate cultivar to help you achieve the desired effect.

If you are looking for a one-plant-fits-all solution to addressing health conditions, you won't find one. Cannabis is an apothecary unto herself. Each cultivar has a different chemical profile and different healing properties. You could spend a lifetime getting to know just a few cultivars of cannabis and how they work under different conditions. Most people don't know what cultivar they are working with, and even fewer know the chemical breakdown of the particular cultivar or what the

cultivar may be good for. The more you learn about the chemistry of the plant, the better your ability to make well-informed decisions about what cultivar to use and what conditions it grows best under.

CHOOSE A CULTIVAR BASED ON THE MEDICINE YOU WANT

The world of cultivars is vast and can be overwhelming. I will offer some recommendations here, but I cannot guarantee that you will find the exact cultivar that I'm using. Every cannabis breeder is trying to sell their product, and cultivars are renamed and rebranded based on what is hot and exciting at the moment. Ultimately, I want you to speak to your breeder or seed

Choosing a Cultivar

Effect	Cultivars	Terpenes
Energizing/Focus	Jack Herer, Lifter, Mimosa, Queen of Hope, Sour Diesel, Super Lemon Haze	caryophyllene, limonene, pinene, terpinolene
Antianxiety	ACDC, Blueberry Muffin, Bubba Kush, Hawaiian Haze	caryophyllene, limonene, linalool, myrcene
Pain Relief	Blackberry Kush, Blue Dream, Sour Diesel, any high-CBD cultivar	caryophyllene, limonene, myrcene, pinene
Sleep	Black Cherry Pie, Granddaddy Purple, Northern Lights	caryophyllene, linalool, myrcene, nerolidol

company, ask questions, tell them what you are looking for, and advocate for yourself.

That said, I will offer some guidance.

Start with a breeder who has been growing cannabis in your region or in a region similar to yours. This is important because you want plant genetics that are well adapted to a growing environment similar to yours.

Seeds are going to be categorized as high THC or high CBD. I recommend getting some cultivars high in THC and some high in CBD. Ultimately, you want to make medicine with a 1:1 ratio of THC and CBD, which you can do by combining plant material from a plant high in THC with plant material high in CBD. Ask for a Certificate of Analysis for high-CBD seeds.

A breeder will know which cultivars they have that will help with the most common conditions that lead people to seek cannabis remedies: energy, anxiety, pain, and sleep. Here are some general rules of thumb regarding the properties of CBD and THC:

* High-CBD cultivars tend to be energizing at regular dosing.

* High-THC cultivars are usually initially stimulating regardless of terpenes.

* High-CBD cultivars tend to be anti-anxiety in general.

* THC and CBD are both pain relievers.

How Many Plants to Grow

If you've never grown cannabis before, I recommend growing four to six plants to maturity.

If you are a person who thinks *more is better* (and I bet you are!), I'd like to take this opportunity to caution you: Those small seedlings may seem exciting and cute and hold oh-so-much potential. But when the labor-intensive step of harvesting comes in September, more plants mean more time than you may have anticipated, especially if you've never grown cannabis.

Think, quality over quantity.

Caring for cannabis plants is not more time consuming than growing other plants in a vegetable garden—you'll need to water them, prune them, and tend to pests. But harvesting cannabis requires more of a time commitment than any other plant you've ever grown. You can figure that harvesting and preparing plant material for drying will take at least 3 to 6 hours per plant. Plan ahead. You may want to enlist some help and/or take some time off from work. Cannabis plants need to be harvested at the time of peak terpene production, which you can estimate. What you can't predict is the weather, pests, and disease pressures that will all affect harvest timing.

Starting Your Seeds

Growing cannabis starts with seeds. You will plant them into 4-inch pots filled with nutrient-rich potting mix. Later, depending on your gardening choices, you can either transplant from the 4-inch pot directly into your garden bed, or transplant into a larger container.

Where do you get seeds? There are a number of reputable seed companies to order from (see Resources, page 130).

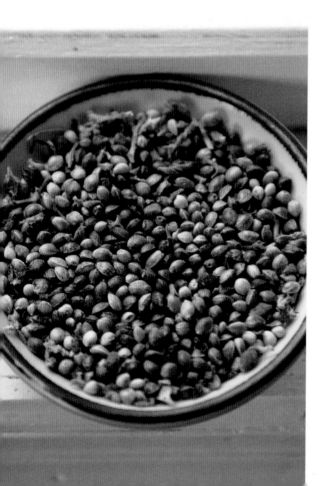

START IN SMALL POTS

I recommend using 4-inch plastic pots to start your seedlings. I know plastic is not the best choice for the environment, so I like to invest a little money and buy sturdier pots that last several years rather than one-time-use pots. Unfortunately, neither of these options is recyclable. Another downfall with plastic pots is that if you let the seedlings go too long, the roots grow out of the holes in the pot edge and then grow around the edge and down to the bottom. The plant becomes rootbound, and the roots have the potential to overheat and dry out.

CLOTH POTS FOR CONTAINER GROWING

If you decide to grow your cannabis plants in containers for their full life cycle, I recommend using cloth pots. These pots air prune the plant roots as they grow—when the roots reach the edge of the pot where there is more oxygen, they will actually migrate away from the edge back toward the middle, which allows them to utilize more of the nutrients in the potting mix. Another plus is that cloth doesn't get as hot in the sun as plastic does. If you use cloth pots, make sure they have handles so they are easier to move around. Cloth pots can be reused, but you will need to get the potting mix and roots out of them, which is a bit more challenging than removing plants from plastic pots.

CHOOSE A NUTRIENT-RICH POTTING MIX

Success in growing cannabis comes down to three basic principles: Start with good genetics, plant in full sun, and plant in the best-quality organic potting mix you can. Potting mix supplies the food the plant needs to grow, so it is worth the investment of time and money. Your goal is to grow plants with minimal input of extra nutrients from commercial fertilizers, so the mix should start out as nutritious as possible for the plants to thrive.

Do not use seed-starter mix. It does not contain enough nutrients to sustain your cannabis plants for longer than 10 days or so.

I recommend a nutrient-rich living mix that will supply your plant with what it needs through its young life in the pot. So, for starting your plants and carrying them through to transplanting out, I recommend a good-quality organic garden mix you can buy by the bag from your local garden or grow store.

Germination

The process of starting a plant from seed is called germination. If cannabis seeds were left on the ground from the previous season, they would germinate. The amazing thing about seeds, all seeds, is that they contain enough nutrition within them to power the growth of the little root into the potting mix and the little stem above ground, and for the tiny leaves to unfurl. All we need to do is provide warmth, water, and air for seeds to germinate.

TEMPERATURE

Left alone, cannabis seeds will germinate when the soil temperature stays consistently above 60°F (16°C) and there is enough moisture in the soil. When choosing your spot for germination, it should be within a 70 to 80°F (21 to 27°C) temperature range. I put my germinating seeds in a warm spot in the house. Light is not necessary at this point. Once the little leaves emerge, the plants are able to photosynthesize and will need to be placed in the light.

CONNECTING WITH THE SEEDS

There are two tried-and-true techniques for germinating seeds. For both methods, I start by putting the seeds in my mouth. (You can put multiple seeds of the same cultivar in your mouth at the same time.) There are two reasons for doing this. First, science. You are providing slightly acidic water from your saliva to the seed and inoculating it with necessary bacteria from your mouth. Secondly, this establishes your relationship with your plants right from the very start. Pausing, with the seeds in your mouth, allows you to take the time to express gratitude for the plant and start your journey of growing and working with cannabis.

METHOD #1: ON A PAPER TOWEL

I prefer this method when I have fewer seeds and especially if I've spent good money on the seed stock. The benefit of this method is that you can actually see when the seed has germinated. The downside is that it necessitates the additional step of transferring the seedling from the paper towel to the pot. Care must be taken not to break the embryonic root from the seed when transferring and to keep your hands clean to prevent introducing pathogens.

1. Determine how many seeds you will be starting, and how many different cultivars. I recommend one cultivar per paper towel package. Up to 10 seeds will fit in each paper towel package.

2. Label a 1-quart or 1-gallon plastic bag with the name of the cultivar and the date.

3. Wet 1 or 2 large squares of paper towel and squeeze out most of the water.

4. Put the seeds in your mouth for 1 minute.

5. Fold the paper towel in half and place the moistened seeds onto the center of the folded paper towel, spaced ½ to 1 inch apart. Fold the paper towel over the seeds and fold the ends up, pushing the paper towel down gently so it comes into contact with the seeds.

6. Gently place the paper towel in the plastic bag and close it up. Place in a warm location (light is not necessary).

7. Check the seeds daily for the emergence of the white embryonic tails. This usually takes 2 to 3 days and can take as long as 7 to 8 days. (If they haven't emerged after 8 days, chances are they aren't going to.) Spritz with water if the towel dries out, but it really shouldn't if it's in a closed plastic bag. Once the tail has emerged, your seedling is ready to go into the potting mix and will be looking for light.

8. Get your 4-inch pots filled and ready. Once the mix is in the pot, use the end of a pen to create a hole for the seedling to go into. The depth should be twice the height of the seedling. This is not very deep, approximately ¼ inch.

9. Using washed hands or a clean tweezers, gently grasp the seedling and transfer it to the pot. Gently cover with potting mix.

10. Using a spray bottle or a measuring cup, *gently* water in the seedling. You can make the pour gentle enough by having the pour height be very short—get the measuring cup close to the potting mix. You need only enough water to surround the seedling with potting mix.

11. You can expect to see the stem and the cotyledons (first little round leaves) to emerge within 1 to 3 days of this first transplant.

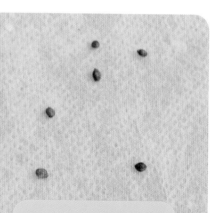

If you start seeds on a paper towel, you can actually see when they have germinated.

METHOD #2: DIRECTLY INTO POTS

This method is great if you have a lot of seeds and want to save time, as it eliminates the step of transferring seedlings from a paper towel to a pot. The downside is that you can't quickly see if the seed has germinated. I have an equal success rate with this method as I do with the paper-towel method.

1. Put the seeds in your mouth for at least 1 minute.

2. Get your 4-inch pots filled with your high-quality organic garden mix.

3. Create a little hole in the mix with the end of a pen, approximately ¼ inch deep. Place a moistened seed into the hole and gently cover with potting mix.

4. Water the seed either by spritzing with a spray bottle or gently pouring with a measuring cup close to the mix.

5. In the coming days, if the mix dries out, spritz with a water bottle.

6. Expect to see the emerging seedling in 3 to 7 days.

A note about labeling: Even if you think you'll be able to remember, label everything! Label more than once. Label the plastic bag you start your seeds in, label every single pot. Permanent markers are your friends. You can buy color-coded plant labels, wooden craft sticks from the store, or put masking tape directly on the pot itself. Whatever it takes, label it!

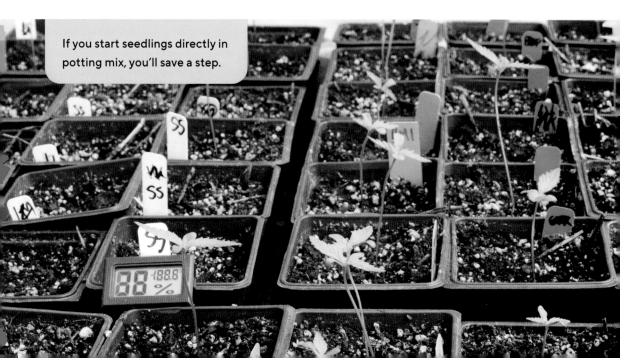

If you start seedlings directly in potting mix, you'll save a step.

Caring for Seedlings

You've successfully germinated your seeds! They've popped their little cotyledon heads up and are starting to put down roots. Now what? For the next 2 to 3 weeks, your little seed babies will be growing roots out of the little white tail (officially called the root embryo) you saw if you started your seeds on a paper towel.

Move your seedlings into a sunny spot or under a low-intensity grow light like a T5 full-spectrum grow light with a kelvin range of 6500, not the high-powered lights intended for indoor growing of cannabis.

ENCOURAGING HEALTHY ROOTS

Establishing strong roots is important. Roots feed the plants so they can grow leaves. Later, when you put your plants in the ground, the roots will communicate with a network of fungal threads (mycelium), bacteria, and the food web below the surface of the soil. This crucial and healthy relationship allows for the exchange of nutrients between the potting mix and your plant. Plants make sugar from the sun and carbon dioxide; they use some of it to build their internal structures and some of it they feed to the soil web in exchange for other nutrients. The more roots, the more exchange, and the bigger and healthier your plants. Simply put, healthy roots equal healthy plants.

WATER IN PROPORTION TO PLANT SIZE

Water your plants to encourage healthy root growth. If you water too much, rootlets are deprived of oxygen and the plant will droop and the leaves will start to turn yellow. Water too little, and the rootlets will dry out and die back and droop. Yes, drooping occurs in both extremes.

The amount of water you add to the pot should be in direct proportion to the size of the roots. The more roots, the more water. Cannabis does not like wet feet; it likes well-watered and well-drained medium. Early on, we are so eager we tend

This healthy seedling shows the smooth cotyledons and the ridged first true leaves.

to over-water. My mantra is: Leave them along, let them grow. Another common beginner mistake is to over-water early in the plant's life cycle and under-water later.

When your seedlings are beginning their life in their 4-inch pots and have just the cotyledons (baby leaves) or their first true leaves, you want to water just enough for the tiny root. A measuring cup works perfectly. Slowly pour water around the base of the plant, with the spout as close to the potting mix as you can get it so the root isn't disturbed by the force of the water hitting the mix. Use no more than ¼ cup per watering to start.

After you water, let the mix dry out. It may take 2, 3, or even 4 days. Pick up your pots daily and start to get a feel for how heavy a wet pot and a dry pot are. You can't always judge by how the potting mix looks because while the top inch might be dry, underneath the mix is wet. If the pot looks dry, it feels light, and your plant starts to slightly droop, it's time to water again.

As the plant develops more above-ground growth and consequently more roots, you can increase the amount of water you use at each watering, but you still want to let the potting mix dry out almost completely between waterings. Cannabis plants will show you how little they like over-watering by drooping, turning yellow, and stunting their growth.

TROUBLESHOOTING YELLOWING LEAVES

Yellowing leaves usually indicate a lack of nitrogen. This can happen for two reasons. One is over-watering, which results in the plant being unable to uptake nutrients at the roots. If you've used nutrient-rich potting mix and your plants have yellowing leaves at the seedling or early vegetative stages of growth, it's usually because of over-watering.

The second reason is not enough nutrients in the mix for the plant's growth. If you see a little yellowing in the bottom leaves as the plant grows bigger in the 4-inch pot, it's time to transplant into a bigger pot. But if your plant is still small (just 1 or 2 nodes of growth), yellowing leaves may indicate that the potting mix wasn't rich enough initially. If you've used an organic, nutrient-rich potting mix, there should be enough nutrients in a 4-inch pot of mix to support the plant's growth for the first 3 to 4 weeks of its life.

TROUBLESHOOTING SPINDLY PLANTS

All plants look spindly as their cotyledons are growing out. If they get taller than 3 inches at this very early stage, they are stretching for and need more light. If you are using grow lights, you may need to move the light closer to the plants, but make sure the temperature at the surface of the potting mix does not rise above

80°F (27°C). If a plant starts to fall over, just tuck some potting mix up around the base of the stem (like a volcano) to help it stand up. Once the plants get their true leaves, they will start to fill out at the stem.

GAUGING WHEN TO POT UP

Once its roots have established, your plant will stop growing vertically and will start to invest resources in leaf growth. Two opposing, single, jagged-edged, finger-like leaves will shoot out above the cotyledon and start photosynthesizing (manufacturing sugar from carbon dioxide and sunlight).

The stem will start to thicken as the plant prepares to shoot skyward and make more leaves. Next, you will see two opposing true leaves emerge from the apical meristem. The apical meristem is the main growth part of the plant at the new tips and leaves. You will recognize true leaves because they are shaped like what we know as a cannabis leaf. The spot where each leaf emerges is called a *node*. When your little seedling has at least 4 nodes of growth, you should start to see root growth coming out of the bottom of your 4-inch pot. This means it is almost time to transplant and do the first pruning.

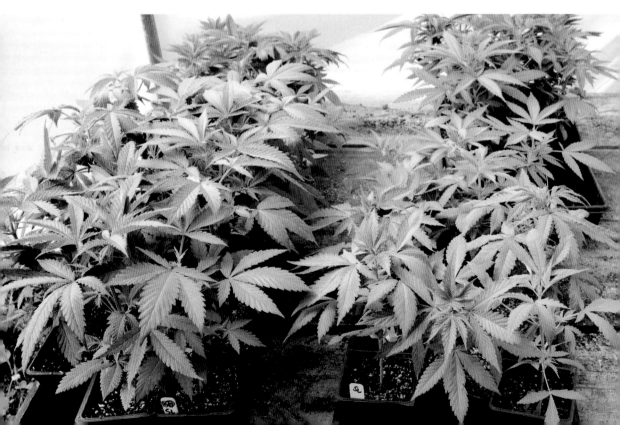

Moving into Larger Pots

Once the roots have developed and true leaves have formed, your young plants will have a lovely growth spurt and will soon outgrow their 4-inch pots. If your plant is a healthy green, its roots are starting to come out of the bottom of the pot, and it has 4 to 6 nodes of beautiful leaves, it's time to move up to a larger pot.

There are a couple other signs that indicate you'll need to move to a bigger pot. Vegetative growth requires quite a bit of nitrogen. When your plant has used up the available nutrients in the potting mix, it will begin to siphon nutrients away from the lower leaves and those leaves will start to turn yellow. If the plant doesn't receive the needed nutrients, it will continue to draw from the leaves farther up the plant and they will turn yellow as well.

INTO THE GARDEN OR BIGGER POTS

So, what size pot should you transplant into? It depends on the climate where you are and where you plan to put the plants for the rest of their life cycle. If the outdoor temperature is above 55°F (13°C), your plant is more than 6 inches tall, and your garden is protected from rabbits and woodchucks, you can transplant from the 4-inch pot right into the garden (or into your largest pot if you are planning to grow in pots). Moving your plants from 4-inch pots directly into a garden

bed or container will require a little more attention to watering, but it is completely doable (see Chapter 2).

If your growing conditions don't meet all the above requirements, I suggest transplanting into 1-gallon pots, still indoors, at this stage. One-gallon pots will allow healthy vegetative growth to continue and give you the flexibility to move your plants outside when needed. Cannabis plants won't grow unless the ground temperature is above 55°F (13°C). It's better to continue to grow them in the 1-gallon pots inside in a warmer environment and wait for outdoor temperatures to rise.

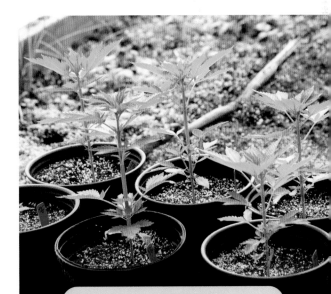

Cannabis will transplant happily into 1-gallon pots while growing, but they won't grow outdoors until the temperature is above 55°F (13°C).

PRUNING IN POTS

Pruning is not essential to growing cannabis. You will still grow beautiful flowers if you don't prune. Left to its own growth pattern, cannabis will grow like a pine tree, where the apical meristem keeps growing skyward, creating more nodes of leaf and stem growth with one leader. This leader will ultimately develop into the biggest flower set called a *cola*. The upper branches (closest to the sun) will also develop big colas. The flowers farther from the sun will be smaller and usually contain less cannabinoids (the active chemicals in cannabis). But I do advise pruning, especially at this early stage. Pruning creates multiple colas and a growth habit more like a bush than a Christmas tree.

The simplest method for pruning is to do it early in the plant's growth cycle, when your plant has 6 to 8 nodes of growth. Many people prune basil when they grow it in a garden, and pruning cannabis at this stage is a very similar process. You can use your fingernails or small clippers to clip down 2 nodes from the top. When you cut the plant here, it will now have 4 tops or leaders instead of 1. They will all grow equally toward the sun.

GIVE SOME HEALING TIME

Every time you cut your plant, it will need to mobilize resources for healing. Best practice is to give the plant 5 to 7 days to heal and recover from pruning before you make any changes like transplanting.

Make the first cut in pruning when your plant has 6 to 8 nodes of growth.

Allow 5 to 7 days for your plant to heal.

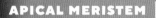

APICAL MERISTEM |—

PRUNE |—

NODE

MAIN LEADER |—

NODE

NODE

NODE

NODE

NODE

On a larger plant, make the cut 2 nodes down from the top.

Hardening Off Outdoors

Your little cannabis babies have been living a sheltered and protected life in the nursery of your home. You have been controlling their environment regarding potting mix, water, and light. Had they been born in the wild, they would've germinated at the ideal time and been exposed to sunlight their whole lives. Also, they would have been exposed to wind, which would have blown around them and stimulated their stems to "buck up" and get strong.

You can manually help them along once they have their second set of true leaves (the ones that look like a cannabis leaf) by gently tapping the stem a few times a day, mimicking the effects of the wind.

The goal here is to stimulate the process of "hardening off." Hardening off is an important part of transitioning your plants from domestication to the ability to withstand the outdoor environment.

STRENGTHENING STEMS

Started indoors, your seedlings have not been exposed to any wind, which is a necessary trigger for the stem to strengthen.

ADJUSTING PLANTS TO THE SUN

As seedlings, your plants do not have the resilience in their stems to stand up to a strong wind. They also need to

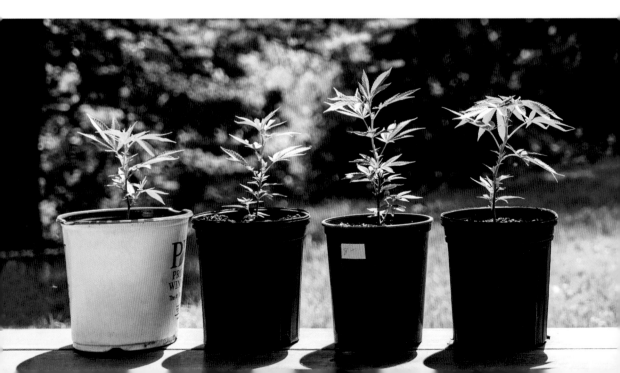

get accustomed to wind blowing across the leaves and potting mix, which will dry them out more quickly than your nursery setting.

Plants started inside are also not used to the intensity of sunlight outdoors. Tiny plants that have been living on a windowsill or under grow lights will quickly bleach out and wilt if you move them immediately into direct outdoor sunlight. To begin with, you should put them outside on a cloudy day or in a spot of dappled sunlight, protected from the wind, for a few hours a day. Gradually increase their exposure time, taking 7 to 10 days to transition them into full sun and wind.

When I move my 150 plants from indoors to my outdoor greenhouse, I try to do it when there are a few days of clouds in the forecast because the sunlight will be less intense. They are protected from wind in the greenhouse, and I can increase the amount of wind they are exposed to by opening the doors. Later, I put them in garden carts and take them on field trips out of the greenhouse for a few hours a day. If you have fewer plants, you can pick them up and move them around, adjusting the sunlight and wind intensity.

Once the stems have hardened up a bit and the plants can withstand the wind and sun, they are hardened off and ready to go. So, let's head outdoors!

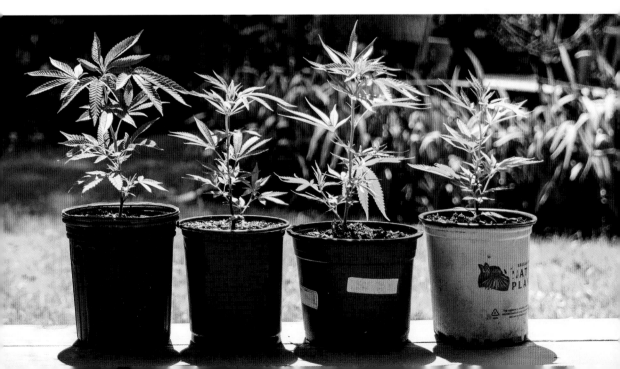

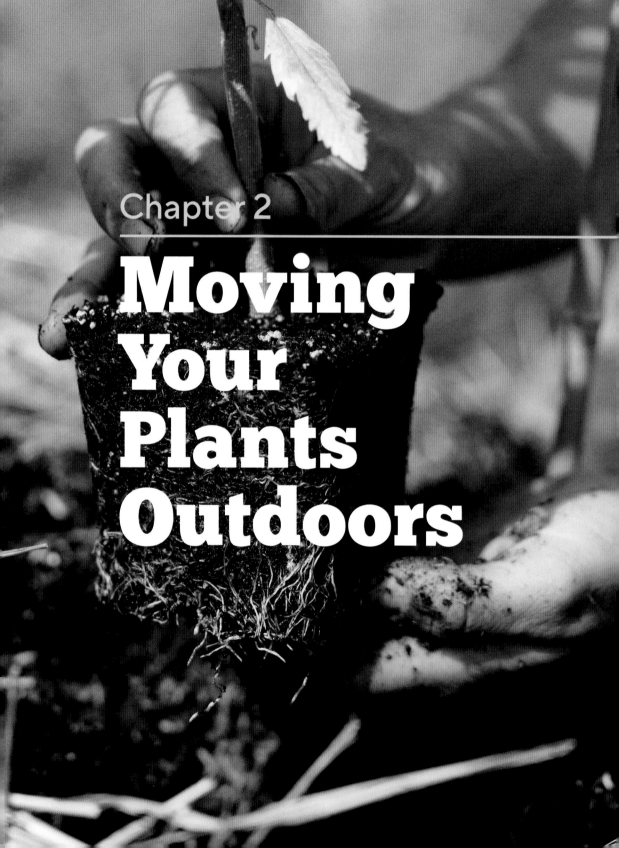

Chapter 2

Moving Your Plants Outdoors

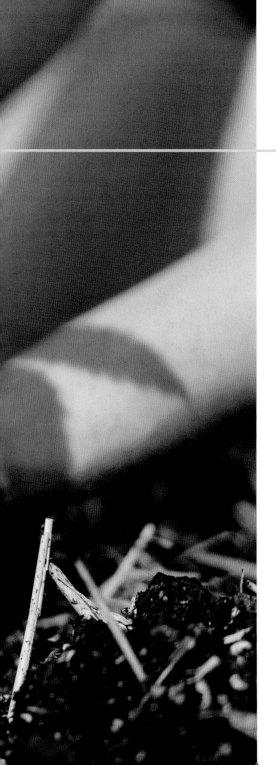

You have grown your little plants from seedlings to babies to youngsters, and now it's time to get them into place for the full bloom of adolescence. They will need a nutrient-rich, well-drained spot in full sunshine so they can do what they were born to do: grow!

Soil Is the Foundation

Soil composition is one of the most important factors in growing healthy and abundant cannabis flowers. Good soil provides the foundation for your plant's growth and well-being. Every nutrient your plant needs must come from the soil. Building a proper soil environment is the foundation of my growing philosophy: Give the plant what she needs and let her do what she knows best, growing and reproducing. If you create good soil, you won't need to add anything more for your plants to thrive.

You can grow beautiful plants in pre-made garden mix with no fancy amendments. I will offer some basic guidelines here, and you can choose what's best for your garden.

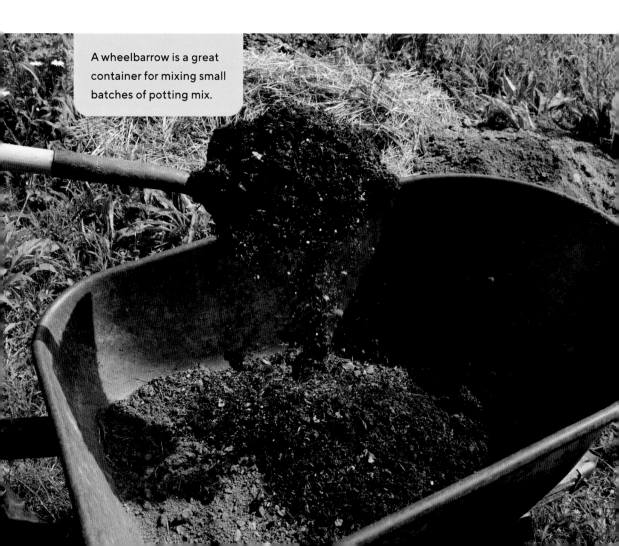

A wheelbarrow is a great container for mixing small batches of potting mix.

GARDEN MIX FOR GROWING CANNABIS

Cannabis requires well-draining, nutrient-rich soil to thrive. If you already have healthy, beautiful soil in your garden, great! All you need to do is wait until the chance of frost is over and the soil temperature reaches 60°F (16°C).

Healthy soil is a diverse ecosystem of microorganisms, including bacteria, fungi, and protozoa, along with insects and worms, that foster a regenerative cycle of nutrients for themselves and the plants growing in the soil. These critters are the foundational component for keeping the entire network healthy. We can help support a healthy ecosystem by providing the right conditions for them to thrive. When the soil network works well, it requires minimal input from us, allows the plant to take in the nutrients it needs, and protects the plant from pathogens. White threadlike mycelium under the surface of the soil is a good indication of a healthy ecosystem.

BUY PREMADE GARDEN MIX

If you are fairly new to gardening, or to cannabis gardening, I recommend buying a premade garden mix. The benefit of a premade mix is that it's already blended and all you need to do is open the bag and pour the mix into pots or raised beds.

It is relatively inexpensive. The range in price depends on the quality of ingredients used and your local market. You can almost always get a discount if you buy in bulk. Good-quality mix is worth the money, and you save the time and effort of making it.

At your local garden supply store, ask what they have available for heavy-feeding plants. If it's legal in your state, you can tell them you're growing high-CBD cannabis or hemp. Always ask what kind of fertilizer is included in the bag of garden mix. Organic is the best option. You want to stay away from salt-based fertilizers. Salt-based fertilizers are cheap and deliver quick results, but they damage the living ecosystem of the soil you are trying to build.

If you have a local cannabis grow store, you can talk with staff about what mixes they have available and what they recommend. Again, tell them you are looking for organic, water-only options (meaning you're not going to be adding growing nutrients to the mix).

Premade garden mixes are rich in nutrients, but not necessarily rich in the ecosystem of beneficial bacteria and fungi that create a truly regenerative system.

Make Your Own Garden Mix

There are benefits to making your own mix rather than buying it premixed. You know exactly what's in it, and it will cost less, especially if you buy the base ingredients in bulk. The downside of this option is that it is more time consuming and requires a little bit of effort to get the ingredients and create the mix before you're ready to put it into the pots.

But don't let that hold you back! Gardening is a lifelong learning experience, and every year we learn something new. You could start with making a few pots' worth of your own mix and comparing it to premade mix, or you could gather with neighbors and make a big batch together.

Recipes for Nutrient-Rich Garden Mix

If you want to try your hand at making garden mix here are a few recipes. These recipes will make 100 gallons of mix, which is enough for five 20-gallon pots. This makes the math a little easier, and you can adjust accordingly. One hundred gallons of mix is approximately half a cubic yard, or 12 bags of premade garden mix.

Once you decide which recipe you want to work with and you have your supplies, pour the ingredients out on a tarp with a 5-gallon bucket for measuring. Layering the materials as you go makes

mixing much easier. Mix with a shovel or fold the corners of the tarp up to move it around. Mix as best you can, and then you're ready to start filling your pots.

None of these recipes are set in stone. They are a starting place for you to experiment with and deviate from. Remember: You can grow beautiful cannabis plants in your garden with no fancy amendments.

My Favorite Garden Bed Mix
This is the one I make for my beds.

* 30 gallons reused premade garden mix or old potting mix containing worm castings, perlite, and other organic nutrient amendments
* 25 gallons mushroom compost*
* 25 gallons composted manure
* 10 gallons garden soil from the ground
* 5 gallons composted sawdust**
* 5 gallons deciduous leaf duff (partially composted leaves) from the forest

  * You can decrease the amount of this one and replace it with equal parts composted manure and old used mix.

  **You could skip the sawdust; I happen to have it on hand.

Abridged Garden Mix

This is an abridged version of My Favorite Garden Bed Mix.

* 35 gallons garden soil
* 30 gallons composted manure
* 30 gallons old potting mix, perlite, or old premade bagged mix
* 5 gallons deciduous leaf duff (partially composted leaves) from the forest

Rich and Expensive Mix

This is a very rich (and probably the most expensive) recipe.

* 40 gallons soil from the ground
* 2 gallons worm castings
* 40 gallons composted manure
* 10 gallons perlite*
* 5 gallons partially decaying leaves

   *If you have sandy or loamy soil, you won't need as much of this.

Soil Amendments

Although amendments are not necessary, you might choose to experiment with some of your plants to see if you notice a difference.

Local Worm Castings

If you can find a local worm farm that feeds their worms regional scraps you have found a gold mine. Local worms contain within their guts local bacteria and fungi populations, which inoculates their poop (worm castings) and then your soil. I'm mentioning regional scraps because the practice of some worm farms is to feed their worms peat moss, a nonrenewable resource, that is ripped up and shipped from peat bogs. The castings from worms who have been fed peat moss won't have the same beneficial effect as those in tune with the local microbiome.

Biocomplete Compost

Dr. Elaine Ingham's Soil Food Web School trains students to make compost complete with all the critters necessary for a healthy soil ecosystem. This compost is different from the compost you might make because bicomplete compost contains the ecosystem of soil critters necessary for a regenerative system. Trained people are available to consult with you and/or offer this compost to spray on your garden.

Korean Natural Farming (KNF) Preparations

Korean Natural Farming is yet another approach to regenerating soil health naturally. A rising network of practitioners is available for consultations and trainings and/or to supply preparations to spray onto your soil.

If You Have an Established Garden

If you already have an established garden your cannabis plants can go into, you may only need to amend the soil a bit, plant some companion plants, or mulch it. Even a well-established garden can benefit from adding some compost for your cannabis plants. Composted manure is your best friend. If you've planted in your beds for many years and have not paid attention to increasing your fungal population or increasing fertility by adding compost or growing nitrogen-fixing cover crops, you'll want to improve the soil before planting.

Add composted manure into the holes you're going to plant in, at least a gallon mixed into the soil of the hole. In the case of cannabis plants, too much composted manure is not a problem. The best cannabis I've seen growing has been smack-dab in the middle of compost piles. You can top-dress as well, which is exactly what it sounds like: putting a few shovelfuls of composted manure on top of the soil and then mulch on top of that. With topdressing, nutrients will take longer to get to the roots than if placed directly into the hole.

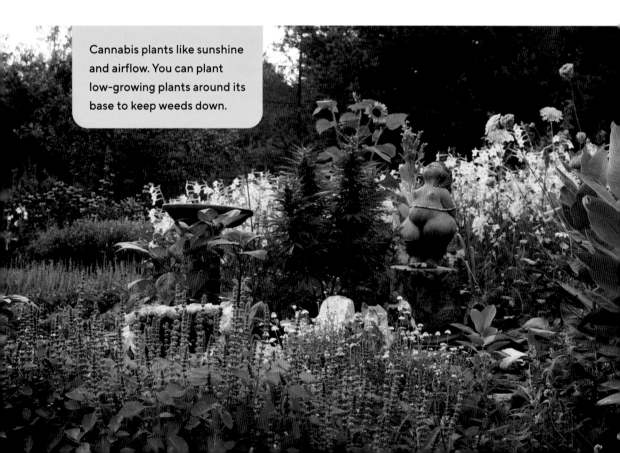

Cannabis plants like sunshine and airflow. You can plant low-growing plants around its base to keep weeds down.

MAKE A RAISED BED

A raised garden bed is simply a contained bed of soil. The goal is to create a deep, wide growing area that encourages plant roots to grow down and outward. You can choose to contain it with wood or not. To create a contained raised bed, you'll need lengths of untreated wood for the walls. The best types of wood are cedar, oak, black locust, larch, or cypress. These are known for their natural rot-resistant properties and last for many years, even in moist conditions. But these woods can be expensive and difficult to find in some areas, and some are not sustainable. Untreated pine is a less-expensive option, but it will have a shorter life span.

Line the bottom of your bed with cardboard, newspaper, or many layers of straw; this will kill the grass. Then layer on 2 to 3 inches of compost, followed by 2 to 3 inches of garden mix you've made or organic garden mix from a good garden supply store, followed by composted hardwood chips (old chips, not fresh).

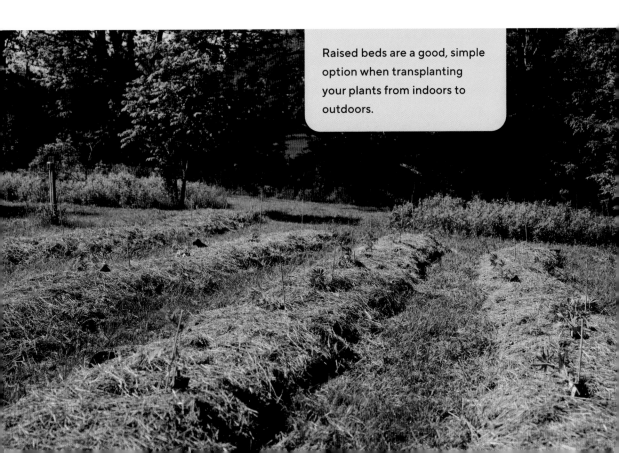

Raised beds are a good, simple option when transplanting your plants from indoors to outdoors.

DIG HOLES INTO YOUR SOIL

Another option besides raised beds is to dig holes for your plants into your existing soil.

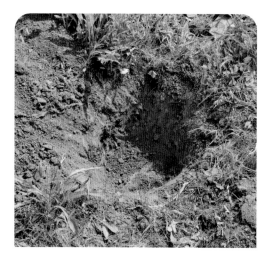

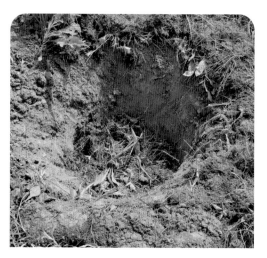

1. Dig holes into the earth 18 inches deep and 24 to 30 inches wide. Keep the soil on a tarp for later.

2. Put the grass back in, upside down, at the bottom of the hole.

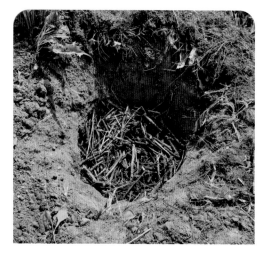

3. Place 1 to 2 inches of shredded composted leaves or small dead sticks or stalks (no larger than ½ inch in diameter) at the bottom of the hole—this will serve as food for beneficial fungus. If you like, you can put in 1 to 2 tablespoons of bonemeal at this point, but this is not absolutely necessary. (This is for a little extra calcium later in the growth phase.)

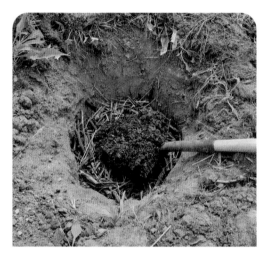

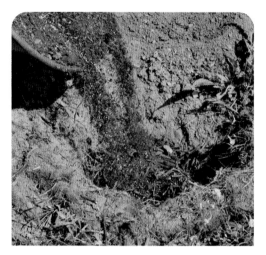

4. Add a heaping shovelful (approximately 1 gallon) of composted manure.

5. Mix 1 to 2 gallons of composted manure with the soil you dug out of the hole and place this in the hole.

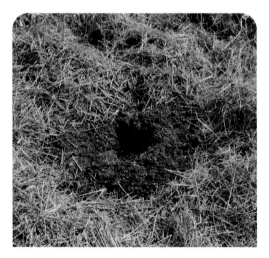

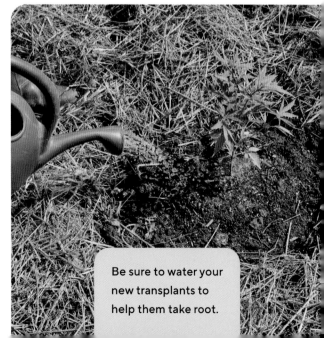

6. Mulch with leaves, straw, or broken-down wood chips.

Be sure to water your new transplants to help them take root.

Putting Your Plants in the Ground

Now you're ready to move your plants from the 4-inch or 1-gallon pots to the prepared location outside.

Plants in the ground will need 6 to 8 feet between each stem so they can expand and grow and so you can move around them. Spacing your plants this way will allow maximum sun exposure on the flowers and allow air to circulate around and within the plant. This will become more important when flowers start to form, especially in cultivars with big, tight buds.

Prepare the spot for the plant to go into by digging a hole with your shovel or trowel. Flip the pot upside down, holding the plant with one hand and the pot with the other, and wiggle the plant and potting mix out of the pot. If the roots are a tangled, webbed mass at the bottom of the pot, you can loosen them a little by carefully pulling them down. Next, gently place the plant into the hole. Your plant should go in deep enough that there are at least 2 or 3 inches of stem above the top of the soil.

If the plant is really leggy, you can remove the lower leaves and plant a little deeper into the hole, burying more of the stem, as you might with a tomato plant.

Tuck the plant in with soil, and water around the edge where the potting mix meets the soil. Watering this way removes any air pockets around the exposed roots.

Composted Manure

Compost made from kitchen scraps is full of nutrients and great for increasing the organic matter in your soil, which benefits the microbes and fungi (I call them the "beasties" or "critters") who live there. However, your kitchen-scrap compost may not have enough nitrogen for heavy-feeding cannabis plants, so I recommend adding some composted cow, chicken, or pig manure. Horse manure is okay, but it tends to be a bit weedier because horses don't digest seeds as thoroughly as cows do. Composted chicken manure is excellent.

"Composted manure" means that it has aged for a period of time (at least 6 months) and broken down so it is no longer "hot," meaning it will not burn your plants with too much nitrogen and ammonia when added to the soil. Fresh, uncomposted manure is too rich and will damage your plants. You could add hot manure to your kitchen compost to fortify it for later use or add it to your garden in fall for the following year's planting. If you have humanure, even better! But that's a whole other conversation.

CANNABIS LOVES SUNLIGHT

Cannabis plants need as much sun as they can possibly get throughout their entire life cycle. The more sunshine available to the plant, the healthier and more productive it will be. At an absolute minimum, your plants need 8 hours of direct sunshine a day. Less than that and your plants will not grow to their full potential. They will also produce fewer cannabinoids and terpenes in medicine made from them.

A sunny location should be the top priority in deciding where to plant. You can always adjust soil quality, but you can't adjust where the sun shines. If you have a perfect sunny spot and not-great soil, you can build a raised bed or grow your plants in pots in the sunny spot.

GIVE THE PLANTS SOME SPACE

Depending on genetics, cannabis plants can grow up to 12 feet high and 8 feet in diameter. This size is the mother lode plant we all dream about. Most will be smaller. Realistically you should plan for plants 6 feet high by 4 to 5 feet wide.

Ask your seed supplier or people who have grown the particular variety you're interested in about the potential size of your mature plants. Equally as important as genetics are the soil conditions and amount of sunlight. Breeders and sellers of cannabis seeds know their plant stock, but they don't know your growing conditions, so any estimate they give you will be approximate. Estimating the size of your plants at maturity will help you determine spacing in the garden and will also help you decide how many plants to grow.

First-time growers often don't believe the plants will get that big or might not

The Plants Do Have an Odor

Cannabis plants have a strong odor. Trust me, it's a bit like having a skunk on your property. When you are deciding where to plant, consider the fact that other people will smell what you are growing. When the wind blows, the smell can carry 400 feet. I live in a rural area, where people cannot see or smell my plants unless they are on my property. The unfortunate fact is that you have to consider the possibility of plant theft late in the season; cannabis plants are coveted and valuable.

have enough space in the garden for a plant to take up that much room. It's better to overestimate spacing than underestimate. When plants are spaced too closely, they compete for sunlight and nutrients, resulting in smaller plants overall and smaller flowers. Plants that are too close together do not allow for proper air movement and can become a haven for mold and mildew.

Allowing for ample space around each plant will also allow you to be able to walk around each plant and prune it. It's important to be able to visually inspect your whole plant all the way around. When I plant seedlings into the ground, I leave 8 to 10 feet between the stalk of one plant and the stalk of the next one.

PROTECTION FROM ANIMALS

Cannabis plants are quite bitter. Most deer, woodchucks, rabbits, mice, voles, or moles, when given other grazing options, will not eat your plants. They might nibble them but will soon forage for sweeter plants. The most vulnerable time for your plants is when they are young. They aren't as bitter when small, and one bite from an animal could remove and damage a large section of the plant. Rabbits will sometimes gnaw on cannabis stalks or eat lower branches if they don't have other food available. My plants have no protection from grazing, and the herbivores in my garden choose other tastier plants. If your garden has a lot of animal activity,

Living Mulch and Companion Planting

When the plants are big enough, you could rely on a living mulch: Plant low-growing plants that don't need as much sun around your cannabis plants. This living mulch creates a green shield for the ground. You could use buckwheat, alfalfa, oats, or yarrow; whatever works best for your growing conditions.

Companion planting can help keep your garden healthy and in balance with the world around it. One approach is to include different-size flowers that bloom at different times, planted among the cannabis plants and around the edges of the garden. All the different sizes and times of blooming attract pollinators, and pollinator insects attract predator insects. Predator insects will complete the balanced ecosystem of your garden and help keep insects that would be detrimental to your cannabis plants to a minimum.

you could put a plant cage around young plants to protect them or put them in a fenced garden.

MULCH IS YOUR FRIEND

Cannabis plants don't like competition early on, so make sure the area where you're going to plant is clear of other plants. Mulching will help suppress weeds.

Once the cannabis plants get 1 to 2 feet tall, nothing will keep up with their growth rate and they will get all the sunlight they need. Mulch also reduces water loss, so you won't have to water the plants as much, and it provides nutrients for the soil. For mulch, you can use a layer 2 to 3 inches thick of straw, hardwood wood chips, or shredded leaves.

Firm the plants into the ground to remove air pockets, then top with a layer of organic mulch.

Growing in Containers

Can you grow cannabis in big container pots outside instead of a garden bed? Yes. If you don't have a large area to plant into the ground or if your soil is contaminated, you have the option to grow outdoors by transplanting your plants into larger pots.

How big do these containers need to be? I recommend at least 30-gallon pots, 40- or 50-gallon if possible. The bigger the container, the more nutrients, the less watering, and the bigger the plant.

Commercial sunshine growers in California grow their plants in 200-gallon cloth pots!

Be aware of spacing between your containers. Cannabis plants potted in 30-gallon containers will grow to approximately 4 feet in diameter, so you should allow 5 to 6 feet between the stem of each plant. You'll need space to get around them to prune and look at them. If your container isn't too heavy, you can rotate it if you need to.

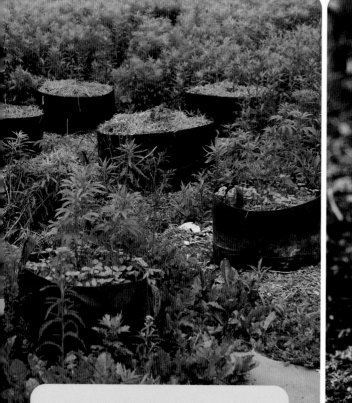

You can grow cannabis in large containers. Companion planting with a cover crop and mulching with straw is recommended.

Cannabis plants will droop if they are over-watered.

Watering Outdoors

In ideal conditions, your young plants would live in rich, well-drained soil; the humidity outdoors would be 45 to 55 percent; the temperature would peak at 84°F (29°C); and we'd have a light rain every few days. Then we could sit back with our iced tea and watch our plants thrive and grow. *Ah, we can all dream!*

But gardening doesn't work this way. While we can't control the weather, we can give our plants nutrient-rich soil and we can determine when and how much additional water to provide.

Cannabis does not do well with standing water around its roots. Well-draining soil allows plants to take up and use the nutrients dissolved in the water without becoming waterlogged. When looking out at my own cannabis fields, I can always tell where the wet spots are by the significantly smaller plants there.

The amount of water a cannabis plant needs is determined by the growing environment and what stage of growth the plant is in. Environmental factors include heat, humidity, and the water-holding capacity of the soil. If your soil is high in clay and holds a lot of water, you will need to water less frequently than if you have sandy soil that drains water quickly.

Seedlings and early vegetative plants require just enough water to encourage root growth but not so much as to overwhelm the roots and soil. If a plant receives too much water, the roots can't get the oxygen they need, and the plant will stop growing. The roots will start to rot and die. Smaller, younger plants need less water than larger plants, as they are not taking up as much water each day. In the rainy early spring, when young plants have little root mass, they will require much less watering than they will in the heat of late summer, when the plants are in their rapid growth stage.

THE GOLDILOCKS APPROACH

Cannabis plants are like Goldilocks when it comes to watering: They want not too much, not too little, but *just* right. Standing water around plants will diminish their nutrient uptake and stunt their growth. Lack of rain and too-dry conditions will likewise diminish nutrient uptake and stunt growth.

An informed grower can look at a plant and determine from the kind of droop whether the plant has been over-watered or under-watered (it will droop under both conditions).

Later in the season (especially if plants are in pots), beginners tend to underwater. It's unbelievable how much water a large plant can consume in a day. In some cases, you may need gallons of water for each plant every day.

Vegetative Growth Stage

Now it's up to the sun and the plant to do their work. Vegetative growth can be astounding! *Vegetative growth* simply means the growth of leaves, stems, and roots. On a hot summer day, cannabis plants can grow 1 to 3 inches! The cannabis plant spends most of its vegetative growth phase accumulating bulk in its roots, stem, and leaves. Vegetative growth is triggered when the plant receives more than 12 hours of daylight. When the day length decreases to less than 14 hours, the plant will transition from vegetative growth to full-scale flower production. Where I live in upstate New York, outdoor plants begin their real growth spurt in June and, depending on the variety, begin flowering in early August through early September.

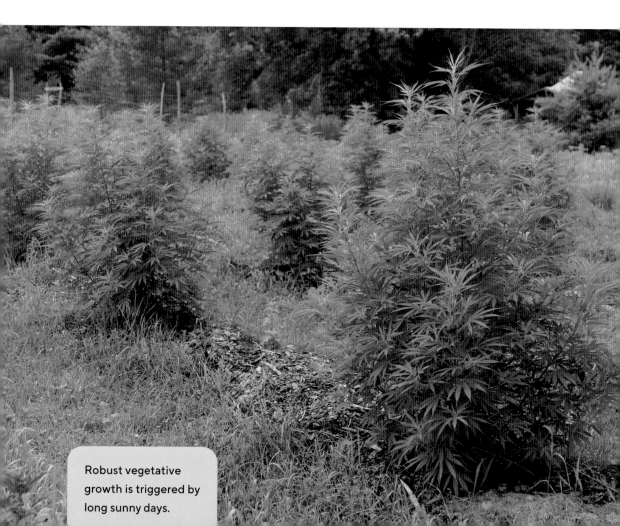

Robust vegetative growth is triggered by long sunny days.

Preflowers

Preflowers arrive during the vegetative growth stage. Typically, we identify male and female flowers during the flowering stage of growth, but some cultivars will show a "preflower" a few weeks into vegetative growth. If this happens, yay! You can pick out the males early. Don't worry, you will be given another chance to find the males in the actual flowering phase of the growth cycle.

During the vegetative phase, the plants' preflowers will indicate their sex. Look for preflowers at the junction of the leaves and the main stem; they will appear approximately 10 weeks after germination. Female preflowers show two little hairs, the pistils. Male preflowers show a small bulbous ball and no hairs. It can be difficult to spot the ball, but the presence of the two hairs is a sure sign of a female plant.

MALES
HAVE A BULB
WITH NO HAIRS

FEMALES
HAVE TWO LONG,
THIN HAIRS

Chapter 3

Flowering Phase

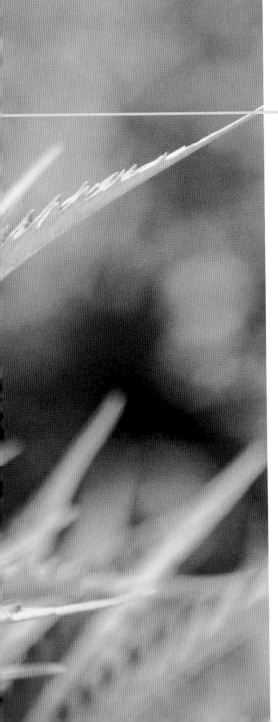

Finally, the part we've all been waiting for! The flowers, also known as the "buds," and the gorgeous, sparkly, resinous trichomes on the flowers house the potent cannabinoids and terpenes that we will use to make healthful remedies.

Flowers Start When Daylight Begins to Wane

Cannabis plants will begin to flower in mid- to late August in the Northeast. They have ended their rapid growth spurt of the long days of summer and are now putting their energy into creating flowers.

Now, the cannabis plant heads into the final stage of its life cycle and begins its work in perpetuating the species. Female plants continue to grow flowers sticky with resin in the hopes of catching pollen carried by the wind. Fertilized female flowers put energy into producing seeds, which, after fully developing, drop to the ground to become next year's plants.

The length of each cultivar's flowering period is genetically predetermined, but all are roughly between 45 and 90 days. People living in northern latitudes should avoid cultivars with long flowering periods because frost can set in before flowering is complete. Reputable seed companies will provide this information (see Resources, page 130).

Identifying Male Plants

Cannabis plants typically produce either only female flowers or only male flowers. Female flowers produce seeds, and male flowers produce pollen (sperm). The one exception is when a plant is stressed. Some female cultivars, when stressed, have the ability to produce a few male flowers (more about this later).

It is very important at this stage to identify the male and female plants and to remove the male plants altogether. Why? Because we do not want them to pollinate/fertilize the female plants and create seeded female plants. We want only unseeded, female flowers—these are called sinsemilla, meaning "without seed." These are the best flowers to make medicine from. Sinsemilla are prized for medicinal use because all of the plant's energy has been invested in producing trichomes—the part of the plant that contains the beneficial chemicals—rather than seeds.

A single male flower can produce 350,000 pollen grains. With hundreds of flowers, each male plant can release hundreds of millions of pollen grains into the wind and into nearby female flowers. That's why most growers remove their male plants as soon as possible. Cutting and leaving male plants in the field will not protect against unwanted fertilization of female flowers. The plants are so virile, the male flowers may continue to mature and release pollen. The male plants must be removed from the growing area and covered.

How to Identify Male Plants

The ability to identify a male plant early on is crucial to prevent unwanted pollination. Males are typically taller than females, and they flower 1 to 3 weeks ahead of females. If your plants are all of one cultivar, keep an eye out for the taller ones; they may be males. This is not a definitive indication of sex, just an early indicator.

Male plants tend to flower before the females. Do not be complacent. Keep checking your plants and removing the males until you have positively identified every single one remaining to be female. I found a very small volunteer male in the field with a single stalk only about 8 inches tall hiding among the females. Sometimes people misinterpret what they are seeing at the top of the plant when the leaves are forming and growing. They may look like little hairs but are actually the leaves emerging. Keep checking in the spaces where the branch grows from the main stalk under the apical meristem (leader).

A fully formed male flower will take a week or so to open and release pollen. Pollen will fall on the leaves, stem, and ground. If you don't see the four-petaled flowers open or any pollen, none has been released yet. And be careful here: If you get pollen on your clothes and then go dancing through the female plants, you may unknowingly pollinate the females.

Once you properly identify the male "balls" of the flower, say a prayer and cut your plant. Either break it down for your compost tea or put the plant in the compost bin and completely cover it so pollen cannot travel on the wind to your girls in the field.

LAB TESTING

Laboratory tests exist that can identify the sex of a plant by the leaf as early as a few weeks after germination. In states that regulate how many plants you can legally grow, it might be worth the money to test your plants early on to identify and remove males from the garden. (See Resources, page 130).

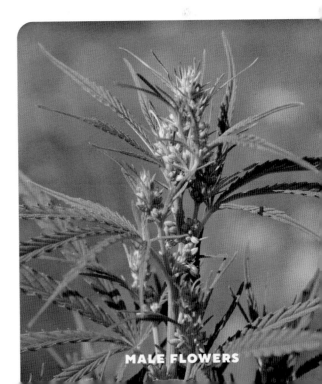

MALE FLOWERS

MALE FLOWER GROWTH PROGRESSION

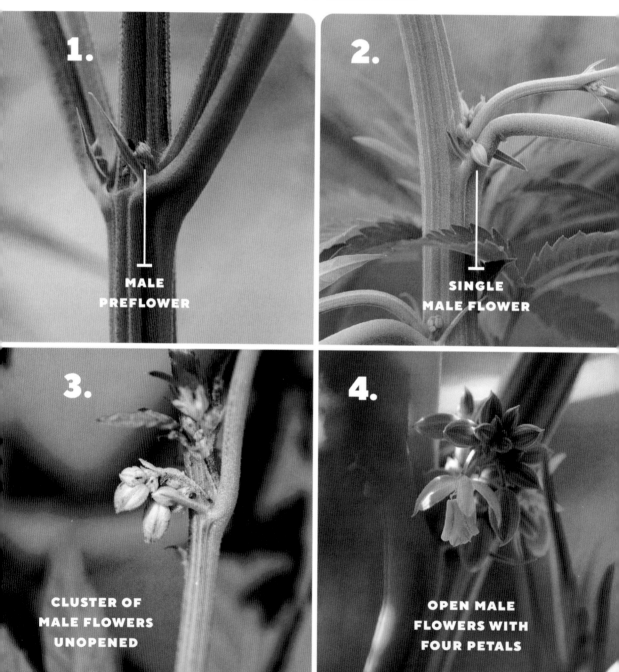

1.

MALE
PREFLOWER

2.

SINGLE
MALE FLOWER

3.

CLUSTER OF
MALE FLOWERS
UNOPENED

4.

OPEN MALE
FLOWERS WITH
FOUR PETALS

FEMALE FLOWER GROWTH PROGRESSION

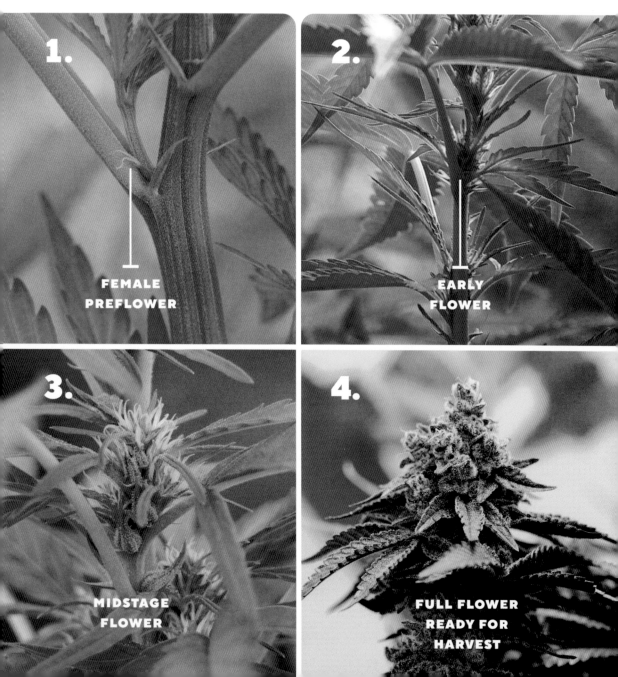

1. FEMALE PREFLOWER

2. EARLY FLOWER

3. MIDSTAGE FLOWER

4. FULL FLOWER READY FOR HARVEST

Seed Saving and Creating Your Own Cultivars

Collecting Pollen

The only reason to keep a male plant is if you want to pollinate some of your female flowers to create seeds for next year. If you are going to collect pollen, you *must* get the male plant out of the garden and in a place where the wind won't blow its pollen onto your female plants (or your neighbors'). Pollen can travel up to 3 miles on the wind, so get those boys in an enclosed space!

Here is my simple method for collecting pollen. When you have identified a male plant, when he is starting to grow flowers but they haven't opened yet, cut the top 12 to 18 inches of the plant and cover and compost the rest of it. Remove the largest leaves from the stalk. Remove enough of the branches so that the entire stalk can fit in a ½- to 1-gallon jar of water without any branches being submerged. Place the jar in a partially sunny window (the plant does not need direct sunlight all day).

To capture the pollen, place a sheet of plastic or a large piece of paper underneath the jar. Over the next 2 weeks, you'll observe the flowers growing, opening, releasing pollen, and dropping it onto the paper. When most of the flowers have gone through this process, you can gather up your pollen and flowers (compost the rest of the plant). Strain the pollen through a tea strainer to collect just the tiny grains of pollen and put it in a sealed, labeled plastic bag in the freezer until you're ready to pollinate.

A word of caution: Cannabis pollen is tiny and light and carried on the wind. Avoid placing your male plant near an open window where the wind can blow it toward your female plants outside.

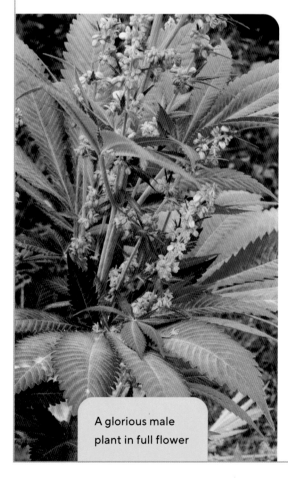

A glorious male plant in full flower

Pollinating Female Plants

The ability to crossbreed plants and create your own cultivars that do well in your specific bioregion is an empowering step in medicine making.

Creating seeds requires pollen from a male cannabis plant to reach the pistils of a female plant. You don't want seeds in every plant in the garden, so you will have to selectively do the pollination work on designated branches of a female plant with a paintbrush or by putting a plastic bag with pollen in it over the branch and shaking it.

Ideally, you will be able to isolate the male plants in an area where the wind will not carry the pollen to other plants—perhaps in a greenhouse or a secluded place downwind from your plants. When the flowering phase begins, wait for at least half of the male flowers to open. You'll start to see pollen falling to the ground at this point.

Place a clean plastic bag over the flowers, close up the bag with your hand around the branch or stalk, and shake the branch. The pollen and some flowers will come loose in the bag. At this point, you can either use the paintbrush to tickle the pistils of the female flowers or put the whole bag of pollen around a branch or two of the female plant. Lower branches work better to keep the pollen more localized. Carefully place the branch to be seeded in the bag of pollen, close off the bottom with your hand again, and shake!

Be sure to label the plant and the branch you pollinated so you can retrieve seeds at harvest.

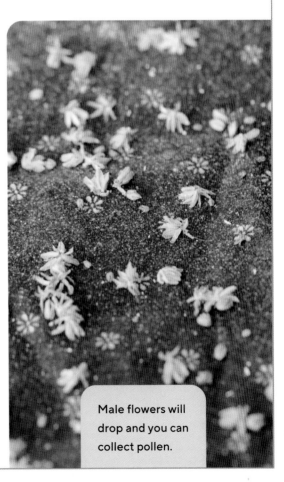

Male flowers will drop and you can collect pollen.

Female Plants

Female plants grow flowers sticky with resin in the hopes of catching male pollen carried by the wind. Fertilized female flowers put energy into producing seeds, which, after fully developing, drop to the ground to become next year's expression of the species.

EARLY FLOWERS

Early female flowers start to look fuzzy with white hairs. These "hairs" are the *pistils*, the reproductive part of the female flower. The job of the pistil is to catch windborne pollen (carrying the male half of the genome) in order to reproduce. If a female plant goes unpollinated, the female flower continues to grow and expand, making more and more pistils and bigger flowers.

It is important to mark your calendar when you first identify the female flowers in the flowering phase. If you know when they start to flower, you can calculate that

EARLY FLOWER

in 7 to 10 weeks the flowers will be ready for harvest.

When the flowers are approximately thumb-size, they begin to make trichomes, the structures of the plant filled with the cannabinoids and terpenes we want in our medicine. At this time, the plants really start to emanate their characteristic smell.

If you want to save seeds so you don't have to buy more next year, now (when the flowers are smaller than the size of your thumb) is the time to get your bag of pollen out of the freezer. Shake it out to cover a branch or two with pollen, or you can use a paintbrush to brush the pollen onto the flowers (see page 47). Be sure to mark the branches you pollinate so you can separate out the seeded flowers for next year during the harvest.

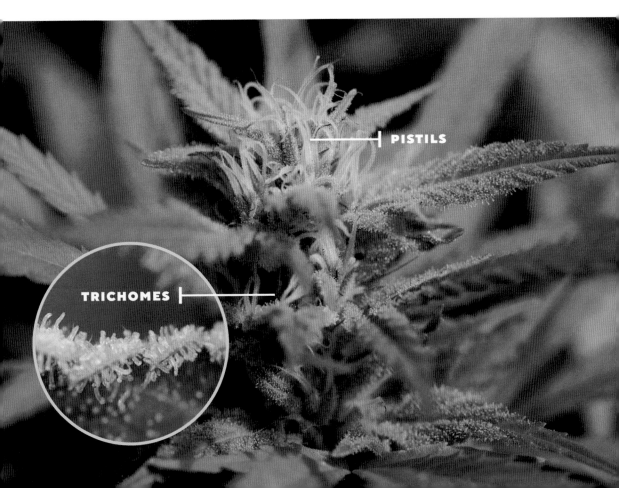

PISTILS

TRICHOMES

FEMALE FLOWER PROGRESSION

For the next 3 to 4 weeks, the flower will continue to bulk up in size and manufacture more trichomes. You will notice that the lower leaves (and perhaps some of the higher leaves) begin yellowing. This is normal. The plant has shifted its energy away from growing branches and leaves and is now making flower production its priority. The plant will pull nutrients out of the big fan leaves—the largest on the plant with long stems—and the branches will stop growing during the flowering phase.

If you have nutrient-dense soil (or you've chosen to use soil amendments), you may not see as much yellowing. Yellowing is okay to a degree. What degree? If more than 25 percent of your larger leaves are yellowing, you may want to give the soil an extra dose or two per week of compost tea or worm castings tea.

Amazing Hermaphrodites

If female cannabis plants become stressed by drought, over-watering, extreme temperature or light changes, or even genetic tendencies, they can take sexual reproduction matters into their own hands and produce individual, male "banana" flowers. This hermaphroditism is quite amazing. If a female plant senses that she will not be able to pass on her genetic line, she will produce these male flowers and pollinate herself! It takes a trained eye to distinguish the single "banana" flower as compared to the multiple male flowers. Banana flowers produce and release much less pollen than male plants, but certainly enough to pollinate the plant that grew it and possibly neighboring plants.

The number of seeds will be drastically fewer than if you had a male plant in the field, and the seeds may not fully mature, but this is not a trait we would want to perpetuate in a seed line.

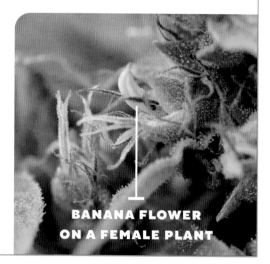

BANANA FLOWER ON A FEMALE PLANT

Medicinal Plant Parts

For making remedies, we use all parts of the plant that produce cannabinoids (CBD and THC are two examples) and terpenes (essential oils). The structures that manufacture the cannabinoids and terpenes are called *trichomes*. These sparkly little glands are found on the flowers, leaves, some stems, and sepals. The female flower herself has the greatest density of trichomes, but all these parts contain trichomes with medicine-making power.

When you grow plants for medicine, it's important to be aware of these small structures because of their vital role in medicine making. In living plants, trichomes are sensitive and can break easily. Throughout the whole process of growing, harvesting, drying, and medicine making, we do our best to preserve the trichomes.

A note about nomenclature here. When I use the terms *flowers* and *plant material* interchangeably throughout this book, I am referring to the mature, trichome-filled female flower with her small, trichome-encrusted leaves.

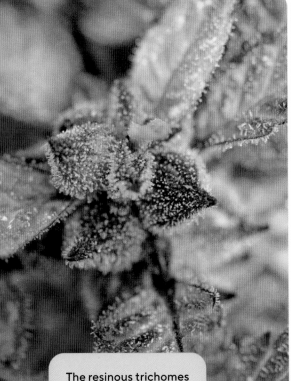

The resinous trichomes are medicinally rich.

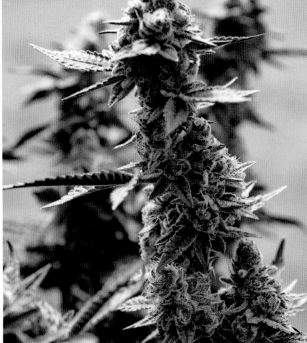

Pruning

The act of pruning accomplishes two things: It increases airflow around the plant and increases the number of big flower clusters (colas). There are many theories on how best to prune cannabis plants. No one particular technique is best. My advice is to consider how much time you have to dedicate to pruning. Pruning takes time, and the more plants you have, the more time you will need. I have a lot of plants, so my pruning tends to be utilitarian in nature.

The other consideration is climate. The environmental conditions your plants are growing in will also influence your pruning. High humidity requires you open up your plant a bit to increase airflow. We will discuss plant issues that arise in high humidity in Chapter 4.

I'll share my techniques with you; they work well and require minimal time. Give them a try this year and take note of what happens. Learn from this year's harvest and try a different technique the following year. Gardening is learning.

Left to their own growth patterns, cannabis plants will grow like pine trees with a tall horizontal stalk that reaches for the sky and lower branches that grow outward reaching to get sunlight. Flowers that receive the most sunlight grow the largest and contain the most cannabinoids.

> Undercutting will create airflow through the bottom of the plant to encourage healthy growth and prevent excess moisture.

INCREASING AIRFLOW

Removing lower branches and larger fan leaves as they begin to yellow creates more airflow through and around the plant. Rainy, humid weather in fall in the Northeast creates a perfect environment for mildew and mold in the dense cannabis flowers. Increasing airflow is one way to help the health of our plants.

If you've ever pruned basil plants to have more "tops," you can similarly prune and train cannabis plants to have more colas. The top cola of the cannabis plant, which gets the most direct sunlight, is always larger in size than lower flowers.

You pruned to create more colas during the early vegetative stage when you snipped the apical meristem and removed the top two nodes.

ALLOW TIME FOR HEALING

Anytime you cut your plant, a wound is created that needs to heal. Healing a wound requires energy. To keep stress to a minimum for your plant, keep your pruning to no more than 15 to 25 percent of the plant's surface area at any one time. This will allow it to heal without diverting energy from growing. Try to time successive pruning with a 2- or 3-week rest and recovery time in between.

DAILY MONITORING

Checking your plants every day is an excellent habit to get into. One of my favorite ways to begin the day is to walk among the plants with my morning tea. I can watch their growth and catch possible problems early on. As you are walking around your plants, you can remove yellowed leaves either with your clippers or by pinching them off with your thumbnail. Remember: Remove yellow leaves (not green, not light green: yellow). Usually, the leaf is turning yellow because the plant is harvesting nitrogen from it, so allow the plant to get all the nutrients it can before removing the leaf.

Size versus Quantity of Flowers

The art and skill of pruning develops with experience. Here's how I like to think about it. A cannabis plant has a finite amount of energy to put into flowers. Flowers at the top of the plant are closest to the sun and will be the largest. The flowers farther down on the plant have less direct sunlight exposure; they will still receive sunlight energy but will be smaller. When you prune the plant down to fewer flowers, it will distribute its energy to the flowers that are closer to the sun and each of the flowers will get bigger. So, do you want 75 big flowers and 25 medium flowers? Or 50 big flowers, 50 medium flowers, and 100 smaller flowers? There's no right answer—it just depends on what you want. Bigger flowers are easier to harvest than smaller flowers, and fewer, larger flowers save you time during the harvest. Or maybe you don't have the time to prune and you've decided to take whatever you get at harvest time.

UNDERCUTTING

Undercutting is an important pruning technique regardless of if you care about the size of your flowers. It is a preventive measure for increasing airflow around and within the plant and supporting healthy humidity within the plant's microclimate. This is especially important to help prevent powdery mildew and bud rot if you live in a rainy or humid environment.

The first major undercutting should happen when your plants have established themselves in their final growing space. (You can prune a few leaves from underneath as you transplant into bigger pots, but this is a minimal intervention.) Once your plants have landed in the ground or in their final pot, give them time to recover from the shock of transplanting. I usually wait until I am sure they've established roots in their new home. If it's a relatively dry summer, I wait until they have put on significant growth of 1 to 2 feet. If it's a relatively wet summer, I'll undercut closer to 1 foot of new growth.

Cannabis plants put on enormous growth during the long vegetative phase. Some cultivars can grow 12 feet in 6 weeks! Even 6 feet in 6 weeks is quite spectacular (that's almost 2 inches per day). The second and final undercutting can happen just when the plants start

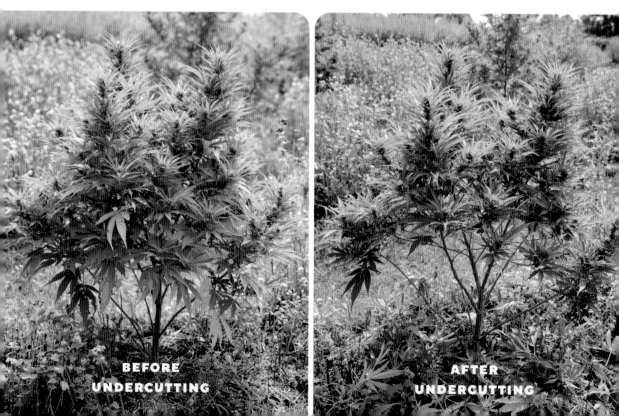

BEFORE UNDERCUTTING   **AFTER UNDERCUTTING**

to flower. At this point, you'll be able to determine which areas of the plant get more sun and remove lower branches that appear smaller and stunted from insufficient sunlight.

BRANCHES AND LARFY FLOWERS

Just like with the second undercutting, this pruning is done by removing smaller branches and flower starts that are so far from the light they won't grow very big. The tiny, airy flowers are commonly called *larfy flowers*. The larfy flowers consume some of the plant's energy, taking away from the net energy available to grow the bigger flowers that are receiving more sunshine. Removing them redirects the plant's energy toward the more viable flowers. The removal of suckers in tomato plants utilizes the same thinking. The advantage of waiting until at least the end of the first or second week of flowering is you can see the difference in growth between flowers that are receiving lots of sunshine and flowers that are not. This makes the job of pruning easier. Typically flowers toward the bottom half of the plant, growing close to the stem, won't receive enough sunlight.

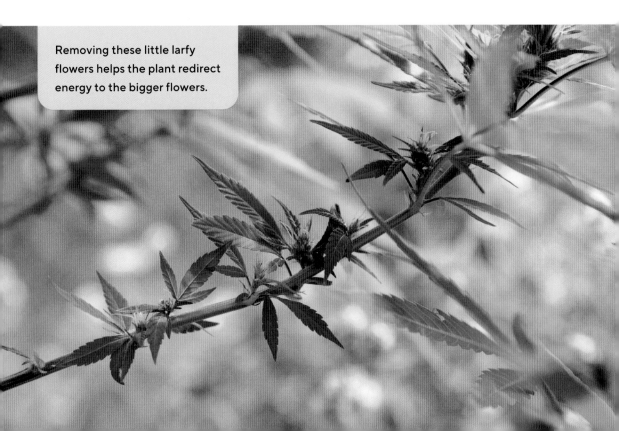

Removing these little larfy flowers helps the plant redirect energy to the bigger flowers.

REMOVING FAN LEAVES

Big fan leaves with long stems grow at the base of each branch, supplying nutrients the branch needs to grow. When the cannabis plant begins the flowering phase, it directs energy resources to the growth of flowers, not branches. Sometimes, if the plant does not have enough nutrients available in the soil, it will pull them from the big fan leaves and they will turn yellow. When this happens, simply remove the leaves when they are completely yellow.

If you have the time and the inclination, you can remove larger fan leaves during the last 2 weeks of flowering even if they are green, especially if they are shading flowers. While this step is not crucial, it does allow more sunlight to penetrate deeper in the canopy and it increases airflow.

When the plants are 4 to 5 weeks into flowering, start removing all the bigger fan leaves with long stems. This allows for more airflow and more light penetration to the lower flowers. More light penetration also means higher cannabinoid content in the remaining flowers. Along with removing bigger fan leaves, you can venture into the main stalks and remove branches in the middle that are not receiving much sunlight.

After the first 4 weeks of flowering, you should remove the large fan leaves that block the light to lower flowers.

If you're feeling adventurous or want to experiment, remove all the fan leaves with longer stems from your plant 2 weeks before you're about to harvest. Some growers swear by this to expose the flowers to more light. Do not remove the leaves around the flowers with short stems (small leaves that you can't see the stems of) since they supply food to the flower. Maybe try one plant and see if you notice a difference. Or even one or two branches on a single plant.

If you look closely, you'll see that the flowers receiving more sunlight will be larger and ready for harvest before the flowers receiving less sunlight. Another way to allow more sunlight to reach the lower parts of the plant is to harvest the top colas first, and then let the lower flowers continue growing another week or so with more sunlight hitting them. This also has the benefit of spreading out the harvest, which you may or may not find helpful.

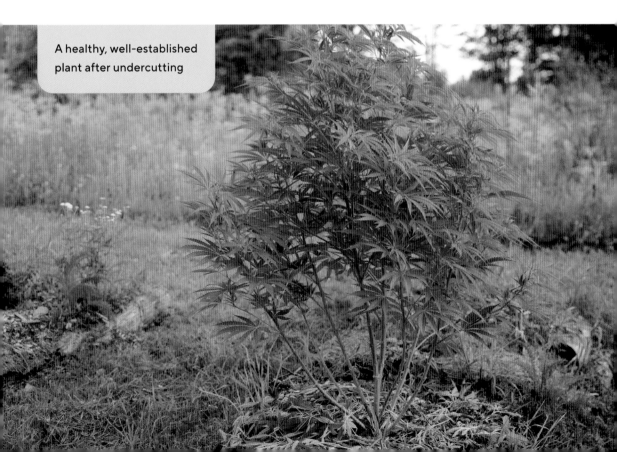

A healthy, well-established plant after undercutting

Chapter 4

Pests, Fungus, and Other Problems

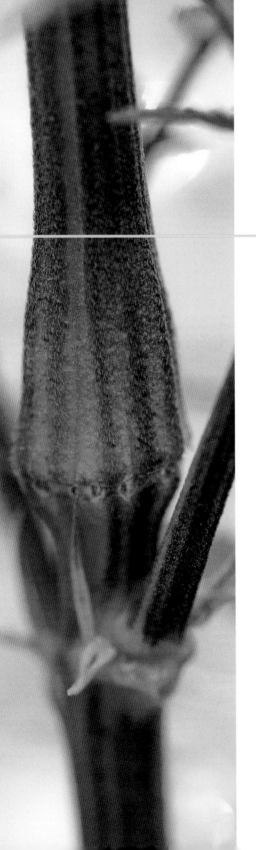

So here you are, it's early August, your plants are cruising along with flower production, and one morning you skip out to your garden and see holes in some leaves—maybe giant holes or small pinprick holes. Or you might see brown spots or little white spots or tiny whiteflies. Or maybe there is some white powdery stuff on the leaf surface. Oh no! You get a horrible feeling that all is not well in canna-land. Don't worry, you haven't done anything wrong. These are typical challenges all growers face.

A Holistic Approach to Pests

Integrated Pest Management (IPM) is a fancy term for a holistic approach to controlling pests. IPM considers and integrates three major aspects: the plant, the environment the plant lives in, and the pest or pathogen affecting the plant. You have tried to create the healthiest environment in the soil so your plants could develop strong immune systems. You've spaced your plants for maximum airflow. Now you can learn how to manage pests so that your plants can thrive.

PROACTIVE PREVENTION

The best way to grow healthy plants with healthy immune systems is to grow them in a balanced ecosystem. Yes, plants have immune systems and ways of fighting predation without us running in with our sprays. Rich soil full of beneficial fungi, microbes, arthropods, and other insects supports the health and growth of plants.

So, rule number one to fight pests is to cultivate healthy soil. Along with healthy soil, planting a variety of flowering plants to attract pollinators will also encourage a balanced ecosystem.

Depending on your specific ecosystem, you will want to educate yourself on regional pest considerations. I encourage you to seek out local resources in the area of pest management, including master gardeners in your area, horticulture extension schools, regional online forums, and your local library, to help build your skills and confidence regarding pest interventions.

If you're concerned about people knowing you are growing cannabis, you don't necessarily need to be specific about the plant. You can talk about the pest and let people think you're growing a food crop like tomato or squash. The same pest interventions apply.

First of All, Perspective

Our ancestors, the plants, are generous beings we can thank for every aspect of our lives. The air we breathe, our clothing, shelter, food, and medicine all come from the green nation. Bacteria, fungi, and the creepy-crawly bugs support the plants, us, and all of life. All of them are much older than we are and have figured out how to thrive in the world by adapting for millions of years before we ever showed up on the scene. So, let's begin thinking about pest management from our right size and place in the world we share with all living things.

POTENTIAL PROBLEMS

If you live in an agricultural area or in an area where people are growing hemp, corn, or hops, you may encounter European corn borers and hemp borers. If you've noticed powdery mildew on your squash, melon, or cucumber plants or on your comfrey or other herbs, you may also be prone to getting it on your cannabis plants. And if you've heard any other cannabis growers in your area complaining of bud rot, you should know that it is caused by a type of fungus known as *Botrytis cinerea* and often results from poor air circulation, densely packed flowers late in the season, late-season rain, or too much humidity.

NOT ALL BUGS ARE BAD

Just because there are bugs on your plant doesn't mean they are dangerous or will harm your harvest. They may be beneficial insects, protecting your plant. Do you see damage on the leaves? If not, leave them be. Also, consider this: Maybe allowing a few bugs to nibble on the plants will stimulate the plant to defend itself. Perhaps this exposure is part of building the health of the plant.

BENEFICIAL INSECTS

Please, do not buy ladybugs. Contrary to popular belief, they are not the best predators. Ladybugs that are available to purchase are wild-harvested, their populations are declining, and many of them end up starving to death before they even get to you. Planting a variety of flowers around your cannabis plants will encourage native beneficial insects far superior to imported ladybugs.

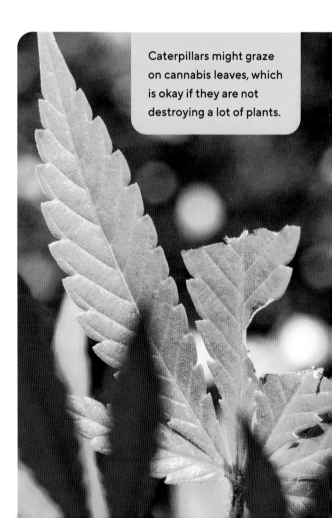

Caterpillars might graze on cannabis leaves, which is okay if they are not destroying a lot of plants.

CHECK THE BASICS BEFORE INTERVENTION

How is the airflow around your plants? Make sure you've spaced your plants far enough away from each other to allow sufficient sun penetration and air movement around them. Be sure you are undercutting properly. Trimming the lower branches, leaves, and flowers will allow airflow at the base of the plant and channel more energy toward bigger flowers above.

Proper watering maintains a healthy plant. You want to water on the ground at the roots of the plant—*not* on the above-ground parts of the plant. Continuous watering onto the leaves will promote mold and mildew, especially in humid environments. It's also the least efficient way to water.

Prevent cross contamination. If you know you have an infection on one plant, be sure to clean your tools before you use them on another plant. This includes your hands!

LOOK AND LEARN

There is a saying that "the best defense is a farmer's footprints." Go out and inspect your plants *every day* for telltale signs of bug damage or mold and mildew. If you see damage on the top of the leaf, flip it over to look for insects. If you see insects, get out your hand lens and see if you can identify what kind of bug it is. Make note of how many leaves are infected. If there are less than five leaves infected on a big plant, you may be able to simply remove the infected leaves and the plant will be okay. If there are more than five, treat early and don't go into denial! The little critters (or it might be fungal spores) reproduce fast, and a small problem can become a big problem quickly.

How Much Is Enough for You?

Personally, I don't think that all the harvest is for me alone. I am part of the ecosystem, and I believe that some of the yield rightly belongs to the life around me. It doesn't bother me if some insects or animals take a bit of my plants.

Here's an interesting fact: Before the advent of modern agriculture, net loss of crop yield was approximately 25 percent. After the implementation of pesticides and herbicides, net loss of agricultural crops is still approximately 25 percent. The long-term damage to the entire ecosystem is not factored into this equation.

SOME SIMPLE SOLUTIONS

You can simply pick insects off your plants by hand. Yep, just pick larger insects right off and feed them to your chickens. Or squish the little ones. Many insects can be removed by spraying them with water; the physical force of the spray washes them off.

You can also pick off infected leaves by hand. This is especially important for powdery mildew and botrytis. Do not put these leaves in your compost. Put them in the garbage to be taken away from your land.

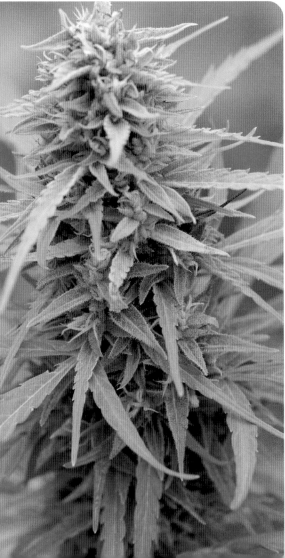

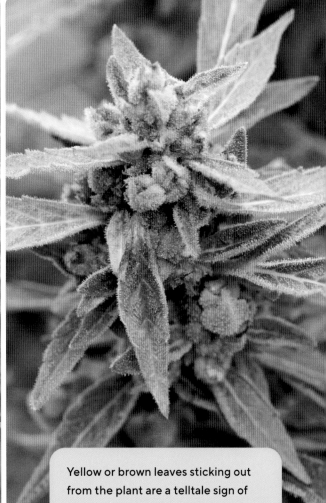

Yellow or brown leaves sticking out from the plant are a telltale sign of bud rot. Check your garden every day and remove any affected flowers.

Spray Interventions

There are various options for interventions, and a few things to consider before you choose to act. Pesticides, even organic ones, will kill more bugs (like bees and butterflies) than just the bugs you want gone. Please research any product, even if it's labeled as "organic" or "safe" or "natural" before you spray it where it could harm bees and beneficial insects. I resist the temptation to spray anything harmful to the ecosystem on my plants.

In general, spray interventions can be applied during the vegetative growth phase without harming the flowers. If you are going to spray during the flowering phase, be sure the product is healthy enough that you would want to ingest it, because it will end up in your medicine. Does it wash off in the rain, for example? Is it promoted for use right up until harvest of food?

Remember, there is a difference between ingesting food sprayed with a substance and inhaling a sprayed flower. Products, even organic ones, usually do not consider inhalation safety. California's requirements lead the industry standards and are a great resource. Buy only registered products; otherwise, manufacturers can add whatever they want and claim it as proprietary information, and you will have no idea what you are spraying on your plants. (See the Resources section on page 130 for more information about insect control.)

When spraying anything on your plants, try it on a small area first to see how the plant reacts. Spray in the morning or evening to prevent burning your plants, which can happen when the sun shines on leaves that have been sprayed.

TOPICAL SPRAYS

Topical sprays will coat the surface of the plant and repel or prevent growth of the pest that eats the leaf or wants to live off the leaf. These pests could be insects, bacteria, viruses, and fungi. Some sprays are intended to be applied directly to the pest to kill it. These include herbicides, insecticides, and pesticides.

I can't stress enough the importance of knowing what other bugs you will be killing specifically with your intervention. Do *not* spray when your plants are flowering. In all my years growing cannabis outside, I've sprayed citric acid once on a few specific plants. That is the only chemical intervention I've ever used. Instead, I've opted to cut out diseased flowers and settled for a decreased yield and a healthier ecosystem.

CITRIC ACID AND LIMONENE

Citric acid and limonene (a chemical found in the rind of citrus fruits) act as an insecticide and pesticide. I use a product called Nuke Em from Flying Skull Plant Products (aggressive name, I know). It kills any soft-bodied insects it comes into direct contact with. I do not use it outdoors because it will kill all insects, including honeybees. I use this product only in the greenhouse, early on, where I can see exactly what I am spraying. I used it for an early spider mite infestation.

You can make your own citric acid spray: Grate the rind of 1 lemon and add it to 1 pint of boiling water. Allow it to steep overnight. Strain through cheesecloth and pour the mixture into a spray bottle. To use, spray on the top and the bottom of all the leaves at the end of the day.

ORGANIC SPRAYS

HORSETAIL. A strong infusion of *Equisetum hyemale* and our native horsetail, *E. arvense*, can be used to kill epiphytic fungi and powdery mildew.

NEEM. Neem is extracted from the foliage and seeds of the neem tree, *Azadirachta indica*. The active component, azadirachtin, is a steroid-like chemical that mimics growth hormone in insects and kills immature insects. It also acts as a repellent to protect against caterpillars, whiteflies, leaf miners, fungus gnats, mealy bugs, leaf hoppers, and some thrips and beetles. It works when the insect bites into the coated leaf and ingests the azadirachtin. It will not harm honeybees, earthworms, fish, birds, or mammals. To apply, follow the

dilution instructions on the bottle. Spray on leaves during vegetative growth and drench the soil for systemic protection. Use acidic water to mix (pH 3 to 7), and spray in the evening. Topically it persists 4 to 8 days in bright sun, and longer when used as a soil drench.

NEEM OIL. Neem oil is a different product than neem. It is an extract of neem seeds that does not contain azadirachtin. It is applied using a 1 percent foliar spray, and is fungicidal, insecticidal, and miticidal. It protects against powdery mildew, aphids, and mites. *This is harmful to honeybees and beneficial insects.*

SPINOSAD. Spinosad is a fermentation by-product produced by the bacterium *Saccharopolyspora spinosa* and can be purchased commercially. It is an insecticide that affects insects specifically and not mammals. The insect must eat the leaf with the spinosad on it. It degrades rapidly in UV light and lasts up to 7 days. It protects against caterpillars, thrips, beetles, and leaf miner maggots. Spray topically every 7 days on vegetative growth.

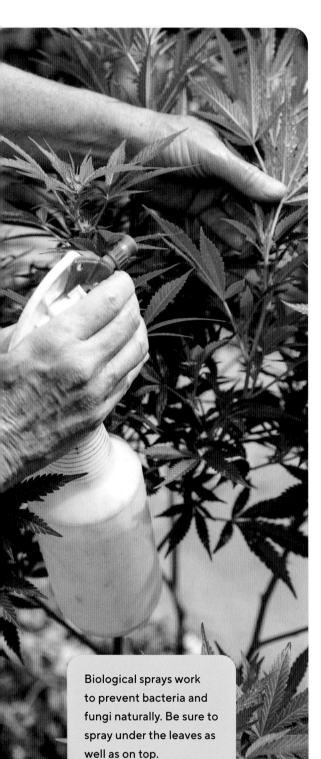

Biological sprays work to prevent bacteria and fungi naturally. Be sure to spray under the leaves as well as on top.

BIOLOGICAL SPRAYS

Biological sprays work in one of two ways. Some sprays are made of beneficial bacteria or fungi that coat the leaf and take up space on the surface so that pathogenic bacteria or fungi can't get a foothold. Others are plant-based extracts that, when sprayed on the plant, stimulate the plant's immune system into action. They are "life based" (biology is the study of life) rather than chemically based.

BACILLUS THURINGIENSIS (BT)

Bacillus thuringiensis is a species of bacteria that lives in soil. It makes proteins that are toxic to some insects (caterpillars and maggots) when eaten. Bt must be ingested by the insect to be activated. It is safe for other insects and creatures, including humans. There are many products containing Bt. Look for ones that contain both the spore and toxins, not just the toxins alone. To use, mix the solution in slightly acidic water (pH 4 to 7) and spray on leaf surfaces late in the day or on cloudy days. It degrades with UV exposure in 1 to 3 days, so weekly repeated applications during vegetative growth phase are necessary for prevention. Bt protects against corn and hemp borers, which are types of caterpillars.

HOMEMADE HERBAL SPRAYS

Here are two recipes for herbal sprays that are easy to make at home for pest management of soft-bodied insects.

Garlic, Onion, Cayenne Spray

This simple spray combines common kitchen ingredients and soap.

1. Combine 4–6 cloves garlic (peeled and chopped), 1 small onion (peeled and chopped), and 1 teaspoon ground cayenne pepper in a food processor or blender and process into a paste.

2. Mix the paste into 1 quart water and steep for 1 hour.

3. Strain through cheesecloth.

4. Add 1 tablespoon liquid dish soap.

5. Mix well.

The mixture can be stored for up to 1 week in the refrigerator.

Fresh Spicy Spray

This one from cannabis growing expert Ed Rosenthal is a bit more elaborate.

1. Add 2 tablespoons of each of the following to 1 quart boiling water: ground cinnamon, ground black pepper, ground chile pepper, dried peppermint, crushed garlic, crushed onion, and dried orange peel.

2. When the mix has cooled but while it is still warm, add 2 cups isopropyl alcohol, 1 cup strong brewed coffee, and ½ cup low-fat milk.

3. Strain through a fine sieve.

4. Add 1 fluid ounce liquid dish soap and enough water to make 2 quarts.

Store in the refrigerator for up to 1 week.

Fungal Infections

Cannabis plants are susceptible to common bacteria, mold, mildew, and fungi problems that also affect food crops. Leaf septoria, powdery mildew, and botrytis (bud rot) are typical problems for a cannabis grower, but they can be prevented and treated.

LEAF SEPTORIA (YELLOW LEAF SPOT)

A fungus that commonly infects cannabis is leaf septoria, also known as yellow leaf spot. The microscopic fungus lies dormant through winter in the surface layer of soil and mulch. Cannabis seedlings and young plants will become infected in early spring when temperatures rise above 60°F (16°C) and conditions become rainy. The fungus then spreads when rain splashes the spores onto plants or as you walk through the field and then brush against other plants.

This is a condition to recognize and treat early, before the loss of precious flowers later in the season. Left unchecked, the fungal infection will cause the affected area to die, then the entire leaf will curl, dry out, and die. Eventually, as the infection spreads through the leaves, it can enter the flowers. The dead leaves and flowers can then become a perfect foothold for botrytis and bud rot.

How to Identify

In early spring, keep an eye on your plants for round discolored spots with a distinct border, ranging from the size of a pencil eraser to the size of a dime. Leaf septoria spots are not always yellow. Depending on the species of fungus causing the infection, *Septoria cannabis* or *S. neocannabina*, the spots can be white, ocher, gray, brown, or even red-brown-edged. The distinct border is the identifying factor. You do not need to identify which fungus is causing the infection because the remedy is the same for both.

How to Prevent

Because the fungus survives through the winter and lives in the upper portion of the soil, a balanced, healthy soil is (once again) the best prevention.

If you know leaf septoria is in the environment, you can add beneficial fungi like *Trichoderma* spp. or beneficial bacteria like *Bacillus pumilus* to your soil before planting. This will help inoculate your plants with beneficial bacteria. Follow the specific dilution instructions on the bottles from the manufacturer and then spray these beneficial fungi or bacteria directly onto the leaves of your cannabis plants. Garden stores or organic farm supply stores online will have these products.

Pruning the lower leaves and branches early on, as discussed on page 52, will help prevent fungal spores splashing up onto the leaf surface.

How to Treat

Remove any infected leaves and any leaves that have fallen from the infected plant.

During the vegetative growth phase, you can use topical sprays that raise the pH on the leaf surface to greater than 8. Increasing the pH above 8 will kill the spores and create an inhospitable environment for fungal growth. I like a potassium bicarbonate product called MilStop, from BioWorks, which you can purchase online. Another benefit of potassium bicarbonate is that potassium is a necessary nutrient for flower growth. It is safe to spray during the flowering phase. Spray late in the day, after the sun is off the plant, to inhibit fungal growth.

Sodium bicarbonate (baking soda) will also raise the pH of the leaf surface. The spray must come into contact with the leaf surface and will need to be reapplied after a rain. To make your own sodium bicarbonate spray, mix 4 teaspoons of baking soda per 1 gallon of water. Mix a fresh batch for each application. This is also safe to spray during the flowering phase.

Spraying alkaline water (pH 10), which you can buy at the grocery store, will also raise the pH of the leaf surface and kill septoria spores.

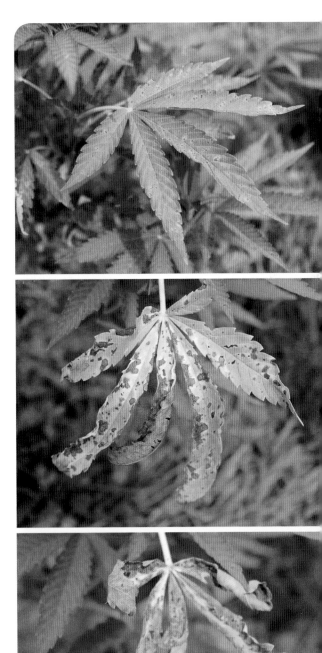

If left untreated, leaf septoria (a fungus) will dry out cannabis leaves and kill them.

POWDERY MILDEW (PM)

Your plants are cruising along, bursting with new growth, perhaps even starting to show fuzzy little flowers. Then one morning you wander out to check on them and you spot little white dots that look like someone dusted the leaf with flour. The fungal family of powdery mildew has come to visit your plants. What to do, besides freak out?

There are a wide variety of fungi that cause PM. They are common throughout the landscape and can infect a variety of plant families including squash, cucumbers, pumpkins, comfrey, bee balm, legumes, nightshades, roses, and cannabis. Powdery mildew spreads through spores that travel on the wind and land on a new host to grow and release spores again.

PM is different from other fungal infections in that it does not require water to spread. PM thrives in warm, dry environments, although it does need short, local bursts of increased humidity on the surface of the leaf to produce spores. These bursts of humidity can occur with temperature fluctuations between day and night, or they can result from consistent overhead watering (lots of daily rain). Plants with dense foliage can also prevent airflow and create microclimates of high humidity.

How to Identify

In the initial infection stages, small white dots will appear on the top of leaves. It looks like a baker dusted the leaves with flour. The infection can progress to infect the stem, undersides of the leaves, and eventually the flowers. Young leaves will be more affected, possibly twisting or becoming disfigured, and turning yellow then brown.

How to Prevent

Grow your cannabis plants in full sun. PM thrives in the shade; this includes small, shaded areas of each individual plant. Pruning and undercutting will help increase sunlight exposure, which will not only help prevent PM but also increase flower production.

Water your plants at the soil level. Overhead watering as a common practice will increase the humidity within the leaf environment.

Healthy soil creates a healthy immune system in your plant, which will help it fight infections. Healthy bacteria and fungi in the soil will populate the surface of your leaf, preventing PM spores from establishing themselves on the leaf surface.

You can also use foliar sprays to inoculate your leaf surface and stimulate the plant's immune response. Biofungicide products that contain extracts of giant knotweed (*Reynoutria sachalinensis*) can be sprayed topically before the flowering phase. Or you can inoculate the surface of your plants with a beneficial bacterium like *Bacillus pumilus* or *B. subtilis*, or with beneficial fungi like *Ampelomyces quisqualis*. These can also be applied after infection.

How to Treat

Check your plants every day. Remove any infected leaves, and any leaves that have fallen from an infected plant. Put infected leaves in a bag and send them to the dump. Do not compost them.

Be mindful of brushing up against infected plants and then infecting the next plant. Clean your hands and your clippers between plants. Clippers can be sterilized with rubbing alcohol.

If the infection has spread so much in a plant that you can't remove the affected leaves, remove the plant from the garden. It is better to cut your losses on one plant than risk infecting your whole garden.

Increasing the pH above 8 on the leaf surface will be effective in killing spores and creating an inhospitable environment for fungal growth. This can be done with homemade baking soda spray, pH 10 water bought at a grocery store, or a potassium bicarbonate product called MilStop, which you can purchase online. (For more information on pH-based treatments, see page 69.)

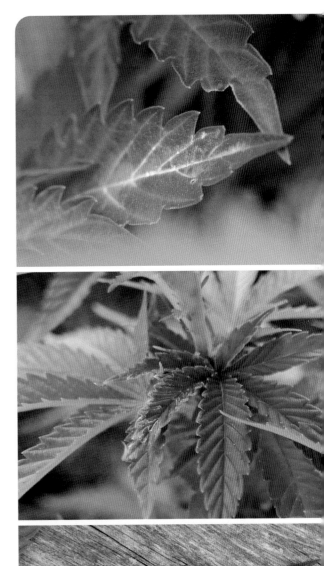

Powdery mildew infections look like a dusting of flour on the leaves.

BOTRYTIS (BUD ROT)

Botrytis, gray mold, bud rot. Whatever you call it, it is the nemesis of all cannabis growers.

It's late August, and your plants have stopped growing upward and are directing their resources to bulking up the flowers. Yippee! Bud density is increasing, the bigger fan leaves are naturally yellowing, and all seems right in your cannabis garden. Then the rains begin . . . and the humidity . . . cue scary music. Rapid flower growth combined with rain and humidity are the perfect storm for botrytis. Prevention and early detection are absolutely the best medicines for botrytis.

There is a genetic predisposition to bud rot in some cultivars of cannabis bred in arid conditions. *Cannabis indica afghanica*, which is called *indica* in the common nomenclature, lacks genetic protection from botrytis. Its ancestor plants were never exposed to the kind of humidity we have in the humid regions of North America. While you can create healthy soil and inoculate the plant's surfaces, it is hard for these plants to thrive in an environment they're not genetically adapted to live in. Their cousin, on the other hand, *Cannabis indica indica* (commonly known as *sativa*), has developed defenses against high humidity and the beasts that thrive in it.

How to Identify

You will see brown or gray flowers that look like they're dead. If you look closely

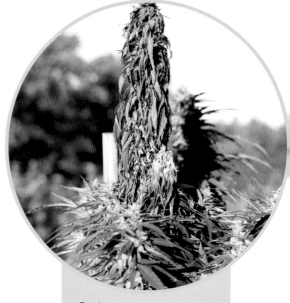

Bud rot can overtake and devastate a whole plant.

at the flowers, you'll see filaments, and if you were to break open the flower you would see what looks like gray dust, which are the spores. I don't recommend breaking open too many infected flowers since you will be releasing mold spores, which could spread.

Another telltale sign is a single brown or yellowed leaf sticking out of the flower. If you see this, go ahead and gently open up the flower a little and look for the fungus. The single brown leaf is what you want to watch for later in the season. It signifies a deeper infection and must be removed. Better to cut out the infected flower than risk spread.

How to Prevent

More than any other problem, bud rot is one you should work to prevent or catch early. Check your plants daily and look for that single brown or yellow leaf. After it rains, go out and shake your plants to physically remove some of the water.

Cut out any mold you see. Be ruthless. Cut all around where the mold is and place those flowers immediately into a plastic bag. Better to preemptively cut out a potentially infected flower than to lose the whole plant. The bag goes in the garbage, not your compost. Then clean your clippers and hands with organic grain alcohol or rubbing alcohol.

How to Treat

Botrytis mold is a fungus, so fungicidal practices (see page 70 for powdery mildew) will also work for bud rot. Be careful when spraying, though. Spraying adds moisture, which creates the perfect environment for this fungal growth. We also want to be conservative with what we are spraying onto our flowers so close to harvest. The safest sprays at this later stage are made from sodium bicarbonate (baking soda) or potassium bicarbonate (see page 69). Typically I don't spray anything on bud rot. I cut it out ruthlessly and wipe down the cut area with alcohol on a paper towel to clean off as many spores as I can to prevent further infection.

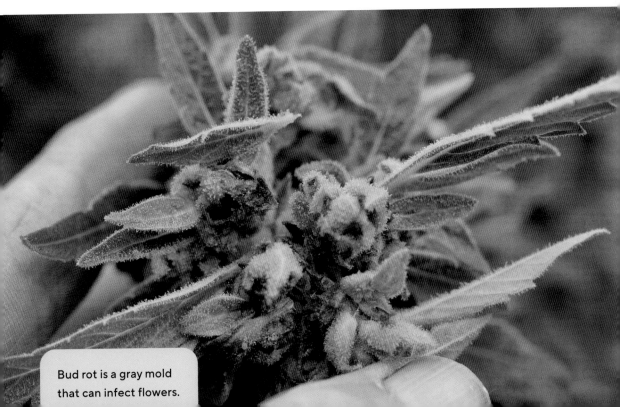

Bud rot is a gray mold that can infect flowers.

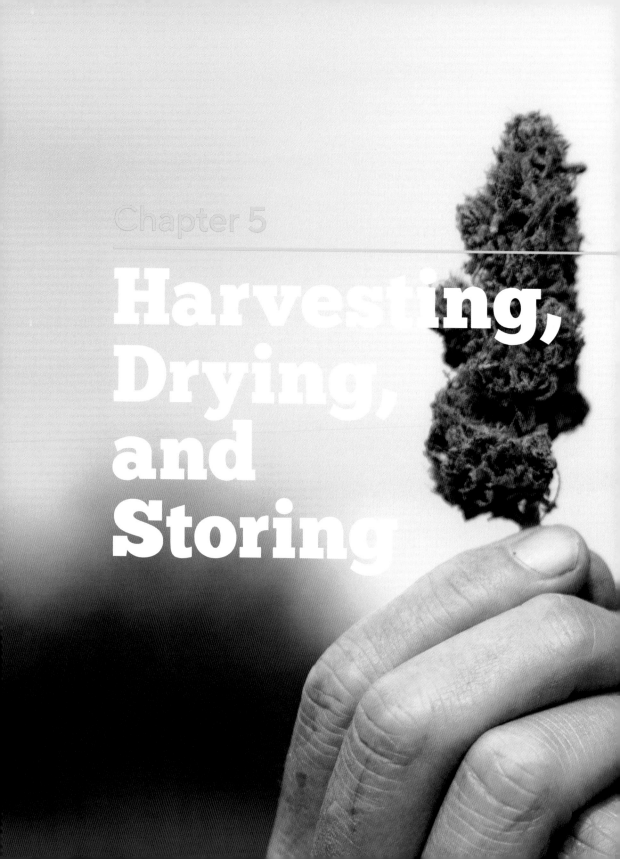

Chapter 5

Harvesting, Drying, and Storing

It's been a long journey with your friend cannabis. Before you harvest, take a moment to thank this beautiful plant for the gift of medicine you will make for yourself, your family, or your community. The generosity of the plant world allows us to live and to thrive in our rich and beautiful lives.

When to Harvest

There are three signs that your cannabis plants are ready to harvest. The flowers will begin to plump up and become firm, the pistils will begin to dry out and turn brown, and the trichomes will change color. A word of caution: A common mistake for beginner growers is to harvest too early, so be patient; you've waited this long, and a week or two more will make a huge difference.

PLUMP FLOWERS

First, the flowers will begin to plump up and develop a roundness and fullness. Start by feeling the colas (the biggest flower on the top of the plant). There is a distinct plump feel to the flowers when they are full. Many varieties get rock hard when they are fully ready. Give your flowers a little squeeze throughout the growing process and you'll start to feel the difference as they get ready.

BROWN PISTILS

The next indication of readiness is when the pistils begin to dry up and turn brown. When you see this, grab your hand lens and inspect the trichomes. Begin to familiarize yourself with the color of the trichomes. Some people will harvest plants when the pistils are 75 percent brown, but a more reliable method is to watch the trichomes.

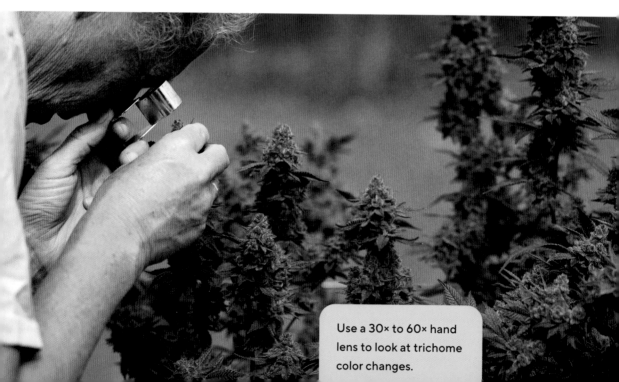

Use a 30× to 60× hand lens to look at trichome color changes.

TRICHOME COLOR CHANGE

The definitive sign of readiness is to watch for a change in trichome color. Trichomes are resinous, hairlike glands that produce cannabinoids and terpenes. They look like sparkly jewels encrusting the flower and small leaves around the flower.

The best way to inspect the trichomes is with a hand lens (not a magnifying glass) of at least 30x to 60x magnification. The trichomes will first appear clear when immature. Then they will turn cloudy. In the final phase, they turn golden. The sweet spot for harvesting is when the trichomes are 75 percent cloudy and 25 percent golden. This is when they are most packed with cannabinoids and terpenes and have not started to degrade. When you see that, it's time to harvest.

Note that clear trichomes are not fully mature. Cannabinoid and terpene levels will be lower in flowers harvested at this point than they would be if you waited until the sweet spot. Medicine made from flowers at this stage can leave a person feeling jittery. Medicine made from a plant with trichomes that are fully golden, on the other hand, can have a more sedative effect.

Trichomes will change from clear to cloudy to golden. When 75 percent of the trichomes are cloudy and 25 percent are golden, it's time to harvest your plant.

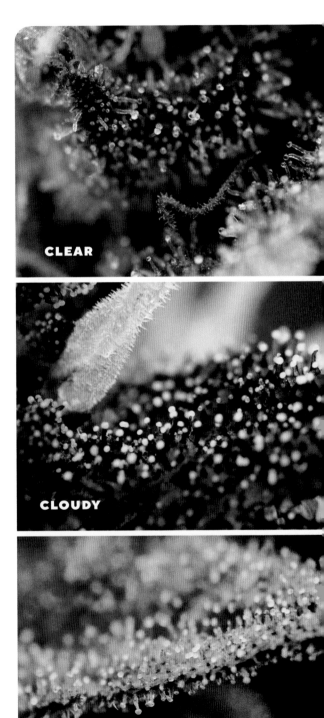

CLEAR

CLOUDY

GOLDEN

Harvesting

I'd like to pause here and say that I have outlined the timing of harvesting as if everything moves according to a textbook schedule. There are many variables to factor in—weather, pests and disease, your personal schedule—and they almost never line up perfectly.

For example, if you see all the trichomes are cloudy, and rain is forecast for the coming week, it is better to harvest a little early (before you see some golden trichomes) than risk getting moldy flowers. In the Northeast, growers are always battling mold. It is important to harvest your plants when they are as dry as possible. Wait until the morning dew has dried off the plants. Harvesting when plants are rain-soaked makes your job harder and sets up a perfect environment for mold.

BIG LEAFING

The first step in the harvest is removing all the fan leaves and smaller leaves that do not contain trichomes. This is called *big leafing*. A good rule of thumb is to remove any leaf with a long stem you can see sticking out.

Big leafing all the fan leaves can take 45 minutes to 2 hours per plant, depending on the size of your plants, so grab a seat, a tasty beverage, and your container of olive oil or alcohol to clean your hands as you go.

One simple technique is to gently hold the flower with one hand and work your way down the stalk, removing the leaves with your other hand. I prefer removing the leaves with my hands rather than using clippers. I feel I have more control and I know I'm removing most of the stems. A gentle downward or sideways tug is

Tools and Supplies for Harvesting

* Small clippers for cutting flowers

* Larger clippers for cutting stalks

* Large (25-gallon) plastic totes with lids or 5-gallon buckets for moving, processing, and storing flowers

* 1-gallon glass jars or large oven bags for storing dried flowers

* Glass hand lens (30x to 60x magnification power) for inspecting trichomes

* Fans for drying

* Herb drying racks, wires, or coat hangers for hanging flowers to dry

* Olive oil or rubbing alcohol with rag for cleaning hands and tools

* Dehumidifier (optional)

usually all it takes. You may even be able to remove two leaves at a time. After you have harvested one or two plants, you will develop your own technique and be a pro.

As you are removing big leaves, look for mold or powdery mildew and use your clippers to cut out any affected parts. Keep a jar of alcohol and a rag available for cleaning your clippers if you need to remove mold. Cleaning your clippers often prevents contaminating the next branch or plant.

The pile of leaves you have removed can either be left where they are to serve as mulch for next year or moved to your compost pile. The exception would be any moldy or mildew-filled leaves. They go to the landfill.

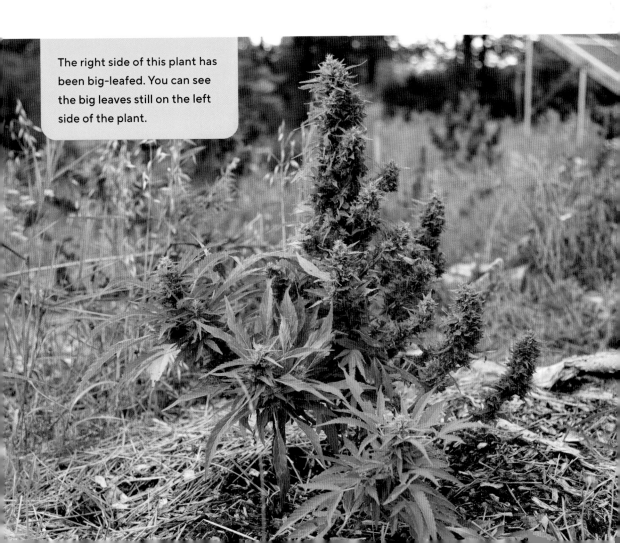

The right side of this plant has been big-leafed. You can see the big leaves still on the left side of the plant.

MIND THE TRICHOMES

Most of the medicine—the cannabinoids and terpenes—in the plant are in the trichomes. The trichomes are relatively fragile, so be careful when you are going through all the steps of the harvest. Being rough or banging your plants around will damage the trichomes. You can't help damaging some trichomes during the harvest process, but when you smell that distinct cannabis smell, trichomes have been damaged and terpenes are being released. And the resin all over your clippers and hands—that's the terpenes and cannabinoids *not* going in your medicine.

Temperature of the flowers also affects the "stickiness" of the resin. Cooler temperatures are ideal for harvesting because the resin is less sticky and stays in the trichomes rather than transferring to your clippers, your hands, or the harvesting buckets.

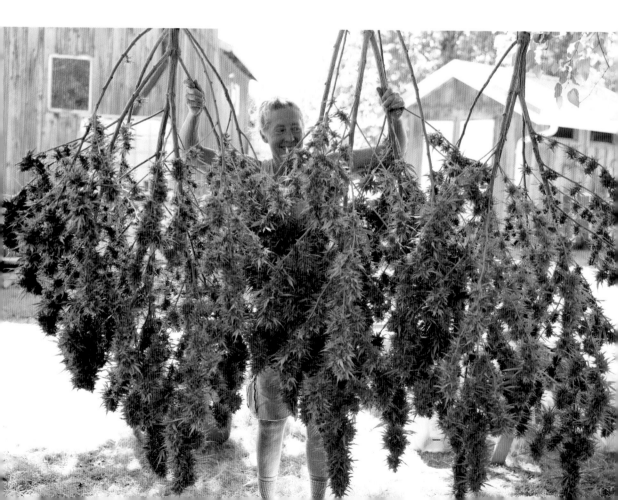

Consider Your Space for Drying Flowers

Guiding principles for a drying location are that the space needs to be clean, have good airflow and moderate humidity, and be relatively cool, with no direct sunlight. Your choices could be in an attic space, a dry basement, a grow tent if you have one, or anywhere in your house if you don't mind the smell. I dry my 30 to 100 pounds of flowers on the third floor of our barn. I put two or three box fans up there, open as many windows as I can, and let the air move across the plants in a cross draft from the open windows. My neighbors know I'm a licensed hemp grower, and I am not worried about the smell wafting out of the barn. If you need to be discreet, you could move your drying indoors. You could also purchase an air scrubber that clears the air, but these can be pricey.

CLEANLINESS. Sweep the floor and allow the dust to settle before you bring your sticky plants in so if any fall, you can pick them up and put them right on the drying rack.

AIRFLOW. Whether you are hanging your plants or laying them on a screen to dry, the space will need good airflow.

You can use a simple box fan. Don't have the air blowing directly on the drying flowers; instead, allow it to circulate around them.

HUMIDITY. Humidity between 45 and 60 percent is ideal. It's harder to regulate the humidity in a barn than in an enclosed room. If you must choose between controlling airflow or humidity, airflow is the more important of the two. In my barn I don't do anything about the ambient humidity, as it's too large a space to control. If you decide to dry in a basement or smaller space, you could use room dehumidifiers to bring the humidity down if need be.

TEMPERATURE. The ideal temperature for drying cannabis is 68 to 75°F (20 to 24°C). Again, this is the ideal. My flowers dry just fine in the unregulated temperature of the third floor of my barn. Do not dry your plants in direct sunlight. Sunlight directly on the plants will cause them to start to degrade.

Drying and Bucking

Before proceeding, you'll need to decide how you will dry your plants. Will you hang the whole plant? Or the stems? Or will you dry just flowers?

There are two basic options for getting your plants ready for drying. You can either leave the flowers on the stems and hang the stems to dry, or you can remove the flowers from the stems in a process known as *bucking*. Here are some things to consider.

Each flower is attached to the stalk by a little stem. The flowers need to be removed from the stalk. You can either do it before they dry and place the bucked fresh flowers on racks to dry or buck them after they have dried.

If you're in a hurry to get the plants harvested and dried, cutting and hanging them on the stalks is a viable choice. Weather may be a factor. Perhaps you only have a window of a day or two and need to get your plants out of the field before it rains again, or maybe you have other crops to harvest now as well. Bucking before the plants dry and hanging them on racks takes up considerably less space, and you get the labor-intensive job of bucking done earlier. Either method works, so the choice is yours.

ASSESSING SPACING NEEDS

How much space you need for drying will be determined by which method of drying you choose. The largest drying racks you can buy are eight shelves, 3 feet across, stacked in a vertical row that occupies

After plants have been big-leafed and bucked, you can place them in a rack for drying.

about 5 feet vertically. This rack will hold approximately 25 pounds of fresh, "wet" flowers that will dry down to about 5 pounds of dried flowers. If you choose to hang whole plants on a wire, visualize a 5-foot Christmas tree hung upside down—that's how much space you'll need for each plant. If you decide to cut your plants up and hang branches on a hanger, figure three to five hangers per plant.

CUTTING AND HANGING YOUR PLANTS

There are two options for hanging harvested, unbucked plants. You can either cut the plant at the base and hang the whole thing as is, or you can cut off individual branches, leaving a "V" at the ends, and hang smaller branch units. If at all possible, big-leaf your plants before you cut and hang; you will save yourself a lot of time and headache by doing this step now. Branches or plants can be hung on a wire or, if you need to save space, hang several branches on coat hangers. Cutting the whole plant into smaller branches, rather than hanging the whole plant, will allow better airflow around the drying flowers.

Depending on the space, weather conditions, and whether you've hung the whole plant or branches, you can expect your flowers to be ready to be bucked and stored in 5 to 14 days. How do you know

they are dry enough? Slowly bend a small branch that's a little bigger than a pencil lead. If it snaps rather than bends, it's ready.

If you are using the flowers to make medicine, you can buck the flowers off the stems at this point and put them in a sealed container with a lid. Jump ahead to the Binning Up section (page 85) for more on how to store them.

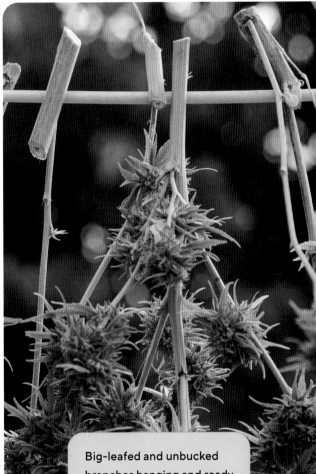

Big-leafed and unbucked branches hanging and ready to be put in drying space

BUCKING AND DRYING JUST THE FLOWERS

The other option for drying your flowers is to big-leaf the plant and cut it down, then find a nice shady spot and buck the flowers off the stalks into bins. After you've bucked a plant's worth of flowers, spread them out on screens or your fancy new drying racks and let them dry. Try to have only one layer of flowers rather than stacking flowers on top of each other. It's okay if they are touching each other on the sides.

The advantage of drying this way is you can check for mold as you are bucking, and this time-consuming step of removing the flowers from the stalk is done.

Once per day, check your flowers and "fluff" them. With your hand, gently move them around so they don't stay in one position during the entire drying process. If not fluffed, they will dry looking squished.

Depending on the conditions of your drying space, drying could take 5 to 10 days. You don't have stems to bend to check in this drying option, but you can feel the flower, and it should feel dry with a little give (not crispy). For you herbalists who've dried other plants, you want it dry, but not to the point that it would crumble if you rubbed it through your hands.

Once they are dry, they are ready for the next phase: binning up.

TOO-DRY FLOWERS

If you take your flowers off the rack or stems and they crumble, they are too dry.

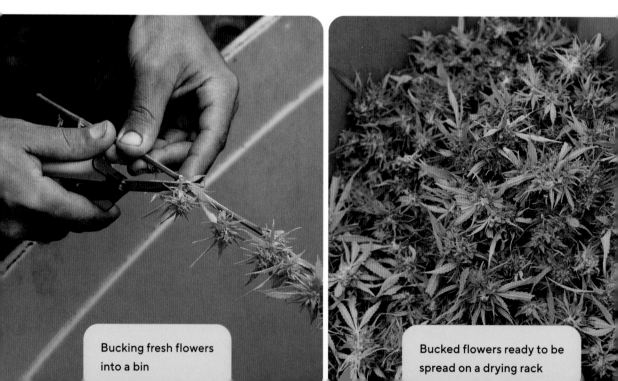

Bucking fresh flowers into a bin

Bucked flowers ready to be spread on a drying rack

Here are two options to help rehydrate them. First, buy a humidity gel pack from a grow store or online and place it in your storage container with the flowers. A less expensive version is to place half a conventional (not organic) tortilla in the container for a few hours to help rehydrate the flowers. Organic tortillas will mold too quickly, so go with the conventional tortillas.

BINNING UP

Your flowers are dry and ready. Now you want to keep them that way. So, you need to put them into sealed containers. The kind of container will be determined by the volume of flowers you have. Option number one would be 1-gallon glass jars with sealable lids, but glass jars are simply not practical for more than a few pounds of dried flowers. You can figure ½ to ¾ pound of dried flowers per gallon jar. If you have a large volume of plant material, your next best options are large oven bags or plastic Rubbermaid-type totes with lids. Look for the large-size bags for roasting turkey. If your grocery store doesn't have them, grow stores will stock them at harvesttime, or you can order them online. Close them up and put them in a bin. When using plastic totes for storage or curing, make sure to tape up any holes you might find in the lids or containers (I've found holes in the handles). A third option is to vacuum seal flowers by the pound in food-saver bags.

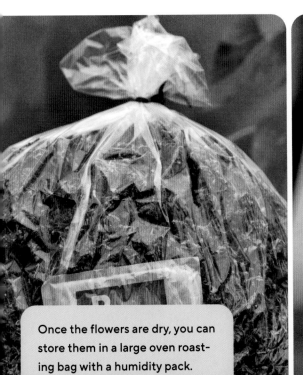

Once the flowers are dry, you can store them in a large oven roasting bag with a humidity pack.

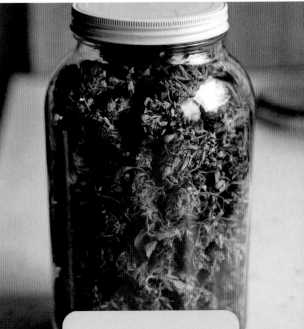

You can also store dried flowers in a glass gallon jar.

Storing Your Flowers

Dried flowers should be stored in a cool, dark place out of direct sunlight. Flowers stored this way will maintain their vitality for at least 1 year. After about 18 months, flowers high in THC will begin to oxidize into cannabinol (CBN). The oxidation process for full conversion can take an additional 2 years. Flowers high in CBD will start to slowly degrade into lower and lower CBD levels starting at 2 years, and may take up to 5 years to degrade.

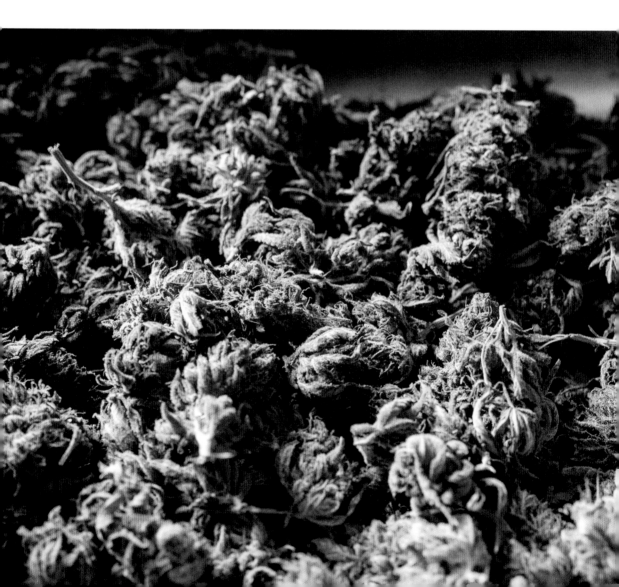

Curing and Trimming for Smokable Flowers

For medicine making, you do not need to cure or trim the flowers. These steps are done only for smokable flowers. I thought I'd give you the information if you want it.

Curing

Curing disperses the humidity completely throughout the flower and allows some of the sharpness of the plant material to mellow. Although it seems like a simple process, curing is an art and is a crucial step for bringing out the fruits of your labor.

If you are going to cure your flowers for smoking, you'll need easy access to them so you can "burp" them two to five times per day for 7 to 14 days. This burping allows the moisture to evenly distribute throughout your flowers, which all have slightly different levels of moisture. It also allows you to check, once again, for mold. When your flowers are dry, place them in an airtight container and open the container two to four times a day, moving the flowers around and then resealing. For the best results, you should cure the flowers for at least 2 weeks; 4 weeks is even better.

Trimming

The smokable flower is just the bud, no small leaves with trichomes. The process of removing the little leaves is called trimming. If you are growing flowers for smoking, you will trim as an additional step. Hanging to dry with stalks is usually the preferred method for smokable-grade flowers. It is easier to recognize when the flowers are ready, and most importantly it allows for better distribution of humidity in the flowers. It also allows you the freedom to trim a little at a time once the flowers and their stalks are binned up for storage. The distribution of the humidity is not as important in flowers for medicine making because we are not smoking the flower and not worried about harshness of the smoke.

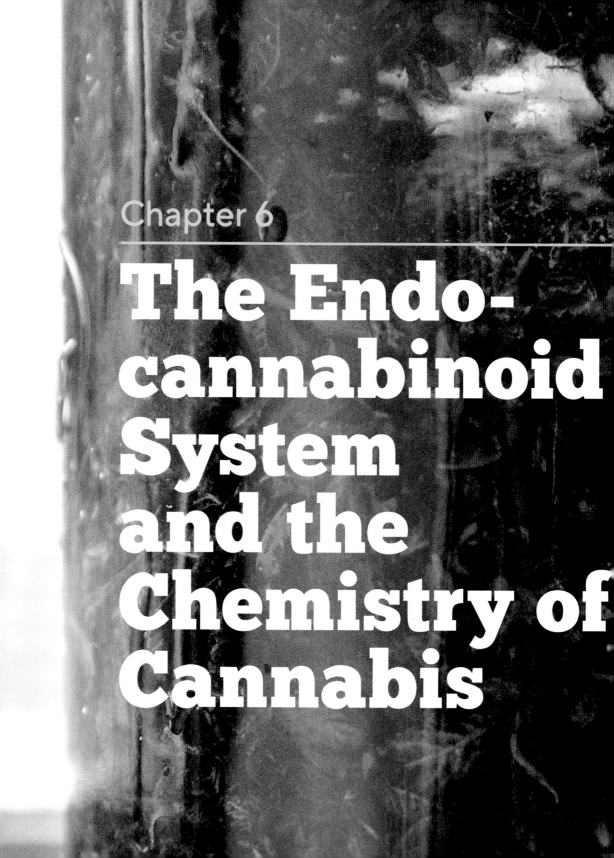

Chapter 6

The Endo-cannabinoid System and the Chemistry of Cannabis

The endocannabinoid system (ECS) is the overarching system in the human body that works with other bodily systems to keep you calm and centered. It is the system responsible for shutting down inflammation. Before you start making home remedies, it is helpful to understand how the chemicals within the cannabis plant interact with the ECS in the body.

What Is the ECS?

The endocannabinoid system (ECS) is a physiological system like the immune system, not an anatomical one like the cardiovascular or digestive system. While we can trace a drop of blood through veins and arteries or track a bite of food through the digestive system, the endocannabinoid system is not as easy to map out. Many of the cells throughout your body can make endocannabinoids or have receptors sensitive to endocannabinoids. The endocannabinoid system also operates like the endocrine system: Chemicals are made by cells, which then travel to and bind with receptors on other cells to produce certain outcomes. The chemicals made by the ECS are called endocannabinoids. *Endo* means "within" or "internal." So, the endocannabinoid system is the system of cannabis within us.

To get a feel for the ECS, let's go on a little journey. It's been a long and tiring day, and the sun is going down. A cold wind kicks up and a driving rain seeps under your collar as you trudge through the gray evening. The sidewalk is slippery, and a car whips through a puddle and splashes you. Finally, you make it to a house. You open the door and walk in, feeling a burst of warmth from the fireplace. You smell a steaming mug of hot chocolate waiting by the fire. You peel off layers of wet outer clothing and sit in a soft chair. Someone hands you the mug of hot chocolate, drops in a few marshmallows, and looks at you with love. "How are you

doing today, my dear?" You are at home; you are safe. This is the feeling a healthy ECS offers.

Our nervous system governs our fight-or-flight response, and it regulates rest and digestion. It also influences important unconscious bodily activities including your heartbeat, breathing, pupil dilation, movement of your digestive tract, and more. The endocannabinoid system operates behind the nervous system and sets the baseline tone for the nervous system.

Questions to ask of the state of the endocannabinoid system would be: Do you feel generally safe and secure? Are you able to relax? Are you curious about learning new things and exploring new information? How are you sleeping? A balanced endocannabinoid system allows us to answer in the affirmative for all these questions.

THE SYSTEM OF WELL-BEING

The ECS sets the baseline tone of well-being in you. The state of well-being is our birthright. When it is healthy, the ECS creates a background signal that "all is well" and quietly hums along as the other systems go about their daily jobs, including the nervous system, circulatory system, immune system, endocrine system, digestive system, and reproductive system.

In a healthy human body, the ECS is activated in response to injury and stress. Endocannabinoids are released to heal the body or reestablish balance. These endocannabinoids affect cognition and learning, emotions, eating, and immunity.

SUPPORT A HEALTHY ECS

We can support our endocannabinoid system through healthy diet and lifestyle habits. Consume omega-3 fatty acids. Limit your intake of refined sugars and unhealthy fats. Maintain a balanced gut. Avoid chemicals that alter ECS function—try to eat organic food and stop using plastic. Manage your stress. Move your body. Get a massage. Limit your consumption of alcohol, caffeine, and pharmaceuticals.

CANNABIS AND THE ECS

The functions of the endocannabinoid system are carried out by endocannabinoids that bind to receptors (CB1 and CB2, if you want to get technical) and create an effect in the body.

The bodily effects of consuming the cannabis plant are caused by cannabis chemicals (THC, CBD, and others) interacting with our endocannabinoid system. These plant chemicals mimic our own endocannabinoids or, in some cases, increase them. They enter our bloodstream through our nose, lungs, and digestive system. Then they travel to and bind with receptors (cannabinoid and others). This binding action causes the physical reactions and sensations we experience as "effects." Cannabis receptors are located in nearly every tissue in the body, so cannabis can interact with and cause changes through the whole body. No other plant shares such a vast and intimate chemical relationship with us.

The Chemicals of Cannabis

The cannabis plant contains hundreds of chemical constituents. I think of these constituents as instruments in an orchestra; they all work together to create a beautiful symphony. Before you begin making home remedies, you should get comfortable with some basic information about what exactly makes cannabis medicine potent and what chemical constituents give the medicine certain properties.

There are three basic categories of chemicals in the cannabis plant we will work with: acids, cannabinoids, and terpenes. Understanding the properties of these different chemical constituents, how they interact with the body's chemistry, and the healing benefits they each bring will allow us to make informed choices about what we want in our medicine and help us make better medicine.

Acids (THCA and CBDA)

TETRAHYDROCANNABINOLIC ACID
(THCA) in the plant functions to protect
against insect predation. When released,
it causes apoptosis (cell death) in the
insect. In the human body, it is an anti-
inflammatory, antiemetic, and analgesic.

CANNABIDIOLIC ACID (CBDA)
is the acid form of CBD. It is found in
live plants and dried flowers. It is anti-
inflammatory and analgesic, and binds
the serotonin receptor 100 times more
powerfully than CBD. The action at the
serotonin receptor may also alleviate nausea and vomiting, anxiety, and depression.
For these conditions, CBDA is the most
potent medicine to make from cannabis.

Properties of Acids

THCA	CBDA
antiseizure	analgesic
antiemetic	antianxiety
anti-inflammatory	antidepressive
neuroprotective	anti-inflammatory
	antimigraine
	antinausea
	antivomiting

Cannabinoids (THC, CBD, CBG, CBN)

TETRAHYDROCANNABINOL (THC)
acts as an insecticide and fungicide in the
cannabis plant. When THC is ingested
by humans, it travels in the bloodstream
and interacts with targeted tissues and
receptors, which is what makes us feel
its euphoric effects in the body. THC can
have many different effects on the body:
It can decrease pain and inflammation,
regulate the immune system, and help us
relax and sleep.

CANNABIDIOL (CBD) protects the plant
from ultraviolet (UV) radiation and acts as an
insect deterrent. CBD has many beneficial
effects in the body. It is an anti-convulsant
and antipsychotic. It increases our own endocannabinoids, helps relieve pain and inflammation, and helps modulate the immune
system and the "high" effects of THC.

THC is commonly characterized as psychoactive and CBD as nonpsychoactive,
but that's not entirely correct. CBD does

affect the mind and behavior. CBD is not an intoxicant or euphoriant, although some people do experience an uplift in mood when working with high-CBD cultivars of cannabis because CBD stimulates production of your own euphoria-inducing endocannabinoids.

CANNABIGEROL (CBG) is decarboxylated CBGA, the precursor molecule for THC, CBD, and terpenes. CBG can be found in hemp fiber cultivars and some high-THC cultivars. CBG is still relatively new to the science community, so we have limited information on its benefits. It is antidepressant, antiemetic, antifungal, anti-inflammatory, antinausea, antiseptic, and has neuroprotective properties. CBG might also be a muscle relaxant and may promote skin cell proliferation. Preparations with CBG in it are necessary for decreasing ocular pressure.

CANNABINOL (CBN) is not found in live cannabis plants but is rather an oxidative by-product of THC. The older a dried flower, resin, or oil is, the more CBN it will contain. CBN will naturally oxidize from THC in our medicines or dried flowers after approximately 3 years. CBN is not an intoxicant or euphoriant. It is anticonvulsant and anti-inflammatory, decreases keratinocyte overproliferation (as seen in psoriasis), and has sedative properties. CBN preparations are excellent for sleep.

Properties of Cannabinoids

THC
analgesic
anticonvulsant
antiemetic
antioxidant
energizing
euphoric
intoxicant
may decrease anxiety
may increase anxiety
muscle relaxant
neuroprotective
sedative

CBD
analgesic
antianxiety
anticonvulsant
antiemetic
anti-inflammatory
antioxidant
antispasmodic
improves sleep
modulates effects of THC
neuroprotective

CBG
anti-inflammatory
antidepressant
antiemetic
antifungal
antinausea
antiseptic
decreases optic pressure
increases cognitive function
muscle relaxant
neuroprotectant

CBN
anticonvulsant
anti-inflammatory
sedative

Terpenes

Terpenes are essential oils in the cannabis plant. Among other things, they are the chemical compounds that make cannabis smell like cannabis. Plants make terpenes in part for protection and in part for communication. Some of the bitter terpenes act as defense against foragers. Terpenes are also sticky and can trap marauding insects before they cause too much damage. Terpenes offer the plant protection against bacterial and fungal infections.

As aromatherapists already know, terpenes are a whole medicinal apothecary unto themselves. Our cannabis medicine is more potent when we make sure to retain as many terpenes as possible. Terpenes begin to evaporate at 70 to 100°F (21 to 38°C).

Terpenes are gaining more attention as important parts of the constituent profiles for each cultivar of cannabis. The terpene profile in a cannabis plant can vary widely, and they are the differentiating factors among cannabis cultivars. Two different cannabis cultivars with the same THC and CBD ratios can have very different healing capabilities. The difference is in their terpenes.

You can submit your flower to a lab for testing to find out its terpene levels. The lab tests are limited since they don't test for all of the 200-plus possible terpenes. Most labs test for the top 20.

For our purposes, I will discuss a few terpenes and the fundamental properties they offer to the variety of medicinal effects of cannabis.

BETA-MYRCENE is the most abundant terpene in fresh cannabis; it is also found in hops and mango. It is analgesic, anti-inflammatory, antimutagenic, antiproliferative, and antipsychotic, and it increases the effects of THC in the brain. Cultivars with higher than 0.5 percent beta-myrcene tend to be sedating, whereas cultivars with less than 0.5 percent tend to be energizing. When I'm looking for a cultivar of cannabis for anxiety or help with sleep, I'm looking for a beta-myrcene level higher than 0.5 percent.

CARYOPHYLLENE is the most abundant terpene in the dried cannabis flower. It has a sweet and woody smell and is also found in black pepper, cinnamon, and clove. It is highly lipophilic, meaning it crosses the blood-brain barrier easily and is highly available to the brain. It also acts as an analgesic, antiaddictive, antibacterial, antidepressant, anti-inflammatory, antioxidant, antiproliferative, antiseizure, antispasmodic, and anxiolytic. Cultivars high in this woodsy-smelling terpene are helpful with anxiety.

LIMONENE is the second most abundant terpene in fresh cannabis; it is also found in high amounts in citrus fruits. It is antibacterial, anticonvulsant, antidepressant, antifungal, and anxiolytic, and it decreases gastroesophageal reflux and serum cortisol (helping with stress). It gives cannabis the citrus smell and, like citrus essential oils, is uplifting.

TERPINOLENE is found in lilac, apple, cumin, tea tree, lemon, sage, marjoram, rosemary, and pine. Some cultivars can be as much as 53 percent terpinolene. It has antibacterial, anticancer, antifungal, and antioxidant properties and is energizing and calming. We can't necessarily distinguish the smell of terpinolene, but I think it's a turpentine smell. When I'm looking for an uplifting cultivar for depression, I look for lower levels of myrcene and higher levels of terpinolene.

Properties of Terpenes

beta-myrcene	caryophyllene
analgesic	analgesic
anticonvulsant	antibacterial
anti-inflammatory	antidepressant
antioxidant	anti-inflammatory
muscle relaxant	antioxidant
sedative	antispasmodic
	euphoric

limonene	terpinolene
antibacterial	antibacterial
anticonvulsant	antifungal
antidepressant	antioxidant
antifungal	cognitive clarity
anti-inflammatory	stimulating
antioxidant	
uplifting	

Myrcene

The presence of myrcene higher than 0.5% within a flower will tend to be sedating. The higher the number, the more sedative (Black Cherry Pie and Grease Monkey are examples of cultivars with a high myrcene profile). Flowers with a myrcene level less than 0.5% and higher levels of limonene and terpinolene will be more energizing. For example, cultivars labeled "sour" (Sour Diesel) or citrusy (Lemon Drip, Tangieland) tend to fall into this category. Cultivars with a gassy smell (GMO, Dogwalker, OG) also tend to have less myrcene and more terpinolene.

Chapter 7

Make Your Own Cannabis Remedies

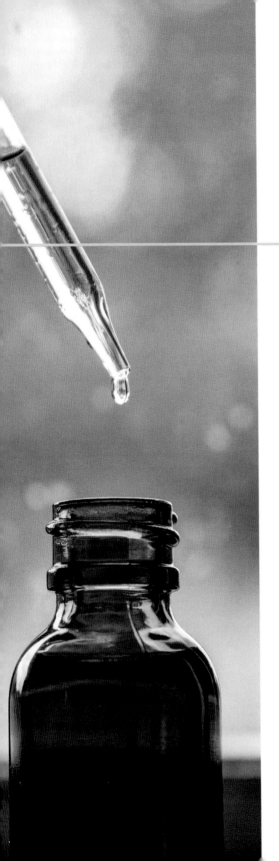

Cannabis remedies can be helpful for common conditions including pain, anxiety, depression, chronic inflammation, and sleep issues. You can make tinctures, infused oils, salves, and edibles. Most people can get what they need from tinctures and oils. Once you make an infused oil, you can then take that infused oil and use it to make salves or edibles.

Dedicate Your Equipment

Before you go out and buy any of the items on the list here, I recommend you read through this chapter, assess what volume of medicines you will be working with, and only then head out to your local thrift store or kitchen supply store.

I recommend having dedicated cannabis medicine–making supplies that you don't need to get spotless for regular use with other materials. As you move into this medicine-making realm, you will start to understand how resinous and sticky cannabis is and how hard it can be to remove the resin from your tools.

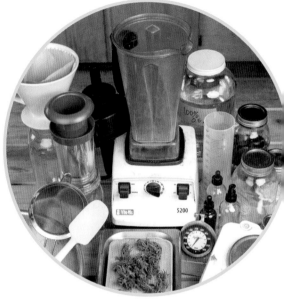

Tools and Supplies

* Mason jars of various sizes (pint, quart, and half-gallon) with lids

* Metal strainer, 1- to 2-cup size

* Cheesecloth

* Rubber spatula

* Pour-over coffee funnel and filters

* Organic grain alcohol or Everclear

* Olive oil

* Casserole dish with lid or stainless-steel steamer pan with lid (optional)

* High-speed blender (optional)

* Coffee grinder (optional)

* Stainless-steel fruit press (optional)

* Salve tins or tubes if you're making salves

* Small dosage bottles (½-, 1-, and 2-ounce) with dropper tops for tinctures and regular tops for infused oils

* Permanent markers for labeling

* Sticky labels or painter's tape for labeling

* Rubbing alcohol or organic grain alcohol for cleaning

Preparing Your Plant Material

At this point, your flowers are dried, with the trichome-rich sugar leaves around them. They've been stored in glass jars or sealed bags out of direct sunlight. They, and you, are ready for the next steps of making medicine. In the jar, they are chock-full of the acid forms of the cannabinoids. If you want to make medicine with THCA and CBDA, you do not need to do the additional step of decarboxylating. More on that on page 100.

Maximizing the Plant Surface Area

When making a tincture or oil, the more surface area of the plant you can expose to alcohol or infused oil, the more constituents will be extracted and the stronger the medicine will be. So, you want to chop the cannabis plant as finely as possible. Think: smaller than a black bean. There are a few simple methods.

My preferred method is to grind the plant material in a blender as you add alcohol. This is good for larger amounts. I've found that using a blender is the easiest and fastest method. A tip on cleaning the blender: Rinse it with grain alcohol after grinding the plant material, then use that same alcohol for making your tincture. You get two benefits in one: You clean your equipment and also recover any resin left behind on the blades or in the jar.

For smaller amounts, you can grind dried plant material in a coffee grinder. You should dedicate a specific coffee grinder for your cannabis medicine, or else your coffee will smell and taste like cannabis.

If you are going to decarboxylate, you can use either method to get the dry plant material smaller before decarboxylating (do not put the flowers in the blender with alcohol). You can also leave the flowers whole for decarboxylation and break them up by hand after they've gone through the oven. If you wait until after the oven, simply rub the dried and decarboxylated flowers between your palms, and then add to your jar for the next step of extraction. Either way works. You just need your plant material small before you add alcohol.

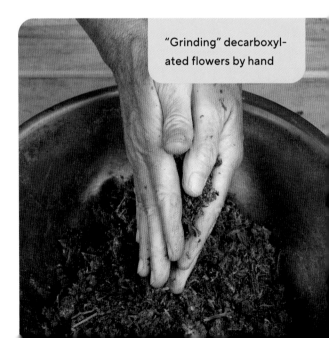

"Grinding" decarboxylated flowers by hand

Decarboxylation

In the fresh or dried cannabis plant, the chemicals available to use for medicine are in their acid forms (THCA and CBDA). If we want to use the neutral cannabinoid forms (THC, CBG, and CBD), we will need to remove the acids.

The process of removing the acid is called *decarboxylation,* and it can happen in two ways. It will occur naturally over time, or we can speed up the process with heat. If you want to make a tincture or oil, you'd have to let it sit for more than 2 years for decarboxylation to occur on its own. This is not practical, so we use heat.

Terpenes are an essential part of your medicine. Although we do everything we can to retain the terpenes, most methods of decarboxylation tend to lose many of them, including big fancy industrial extractors. I've tested mini decarboxylators against the methods described here, and they all resulted in approximately the same level of terpenes in the end. In my tests, there was a 40 to 43 percent loss of terpenes regardless of the equipment used—the decarboxylator, the covered pan, or the lidded mason jar. (The decarboxylator machine retained the most terpenes of all methods, followed by the mason jar method, and finally the steamer pan with lid, but the amount was not so significant that I would invest in a decarboxylator.)

The trick (and the real skill) in decarboxylating is transforming the acid form to the cannabinoid form without overdoing it

and converting THC to CBN (unless that's what you want). If you have had cannabis products sitting around for years, you know that at some point, just by sitting in the jar, they lose potency. You may or may not get the euphoric feeling with aged cannabis, but you will definitely get the sedation from CBN. Some people will try to convince you that freezing cannabis will slow this process down, and it just isn't true. Time still exists in the freezer!

HEAT DECARBOXYLATION

You can use your oven for decarboxylation. The easiest method is to put a 1- to 2-inch layer of flowers in a covered steamer pan or casserole dish with a lid. For smaller quantities, mason jars with lids lightly screwed on work perfectly well for decarboxylating and retaining as many of the terpenes as possible. (And it prevents your house from smelling like cannabis!)

Put the pan or jar in a 250°F (121°C) preheated oven and heat it for 60 minutes for THC and 80 minutes for CBD, shaking with the lid on every 15 to 20 minutes. THC and CBD decarboxylate at slightly different temperatures, but this method will safely extract both cannabinoids. As you get to know your oven, you can fine-tune your method, heating a bit longer or at a higher temperature.

Don't trust your oven's internal thermometer. Use a freestanding oven thermometer to make sure the temperature is

250°F (121°C). Heating above 100°F (38°C) evaporates terpenes; you will smell them evaporating as you heat the flowers. Too high a temperature will result in even more terpene loss, although covering the pan or jar helps retain some of the terpenes.

At the end of the allotted time, remove the covered pan or jar from the oven and let it cool to room temperature with the lid on. Do not remove the lid. Once cool, shake the pan or jar upside down to transfer any terpene condensate from the inside of the lid back to your flowers. Be sure to scrape all the dust (called *keif*) from the bottom of the pan. That dust is the trichomes that have broken off the leaves and flowers. You want that!

MINI DECARBOXYLATORS

You can buy a handy-dandy mini-decarboxylator that will decarboxylate 1 to 4 ounces of flowers in less than 2 hours. The drawbacks are cost and relatively small capacity. They don't necessarily retain any more terpenes than the method described above.

DO YOU REALLY NEED TO DECARBOXYLATE?

If you want to work with the acid forms THCA or CBDA only, no, you do not need to decarboxylate. You can make good remedies by not decarboxylating and retaining all the terpenes. The medicine you make with un-decarboxylated plant material will not contain the cannabinoids THC, CBD, and CBG. If you want the best of both worlds, you can make a tincture of the decarboxylated forms and another tincture with the acid forms and more of the terpenes, then combine the two!

Fine-Tuning Your Method

As you make remedies over time, you will develop your own method for grinding the flowers and standardizing the whole process. If you want to see how well you are extracting and decarboxylating, make a tincture and have it tested. The ratio of acid to cannabinoid will tell you how well your decarboxylation process works. The more THCA or CBDA you have left over, the less decarboxylation occurred and the longer you may need to decarboxylate to increase the amount of THC, CBD, and CBG. After a few rounds of making medicine and testing, you can fine-tune the process. Maybe you'll need to decarboxylate for a little longer in the oven, or maybe go to a slightly higher temperature.

CONSISTENT DOSING

If you want consistent dosing across multiple batches of medicine, a few additional steps can help.

- Grind dried flowers to a similar consistency for each batch. I use my blender for all tincture making (any high-speed blender or food processor will work).

- Weigh the dried flowers in grams before you add them to alcohol/oil for the acid form; or if you decarboxylate, weigh them after the process.

- Measure the strained alcohol in milliliters when you are done.

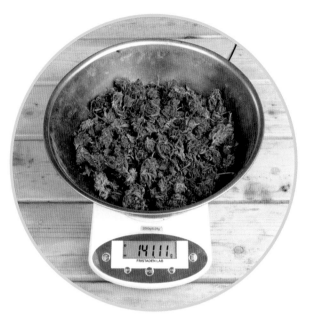

Decide on the ratio of flowers to alcohol and use that ratio consistently. Common ratios for making medicines are 1:5 or 1:10. The proportions are grams of dried flowers to milliliters of alcohol. A 1:5 ratio would yield a more potent extract.

For example, 114 grams of flowers to 570 milliliters (2.4 cups) of alcohol would be a 1:5 ratio. And 114 grams of flowers to 1,140 mL (4.75 cups) of alcohol would be a 1:10 ratio. Knowing the weight of flowers and milliliters of solvent will allow you to calculate dosage later.

Simplars Method

Not interested in all the measuring and weighing? The simplars method offers another way. This traditional method is to fill a container with plant material, then fill the container with oil or alcohol. This usually ends up at around a 1:5 ratio (1 gram of plant material to 5 mLs of liquid).

Tinctures

Tinctures of cannabis are potent remedies for most conditions you will be looking to treat. They absorb quickly into the body (in 10 to 30 minutes) and are simple to make.

Making a tincture is the process of extracting active constituents from a plant with a solvent. It can be as simple as cutting plant material into small pieces, filling a jar with the plant material, and covering the plant material completely with alcohol. Then, as we herbalists like to say, "shake and pray every day" for 3 to 6 weeks, strain, and store in a cool, dry place. Yes, it is that simple.

Although herbalists are taught that cannabinoid extraction takes 3 to 6 weeks, it actually only takes an hour! It's true, and I know that's hard to believe. It really depends on when you need your medicine, because either timeline works. (We herbalists have other reasons for letting the plants sit in tincture for weeks, like the phases of the moon, for example.) Any process that breaks down the cannabis trichomes and exposes their contents to alcohol or glycerin will work for making a tincture.

When making a tincture with something as resinous as cannabis, you need to use a solvent with an alcohol content of at least 95 percent, or 190 proof. Studies done with lower alcohol percentages show diminished extraction rates for cannabinoids. Organic grain alcohol bought in bulk is the cheapest option. Organic, in this case, means it's made with a carbon-based mash such as corn or another grain, potatoes, or sugar. It does not mean that it meets USDA organic growing standards. There are grain alcohols that are made from organically grown ingredients, such as organic neutral grape spirits. Prices for these are two to three times higher than regular grain alcohol. Note that organic grain alcohol is a distilled alcohol and is naturally gluten-free regardless of the mash or marketing.

Some people prefer not to use alcohol for sensitivity or substance-abuse reasons. You can extract using glycerin instead, although it is not as effective at extraction.

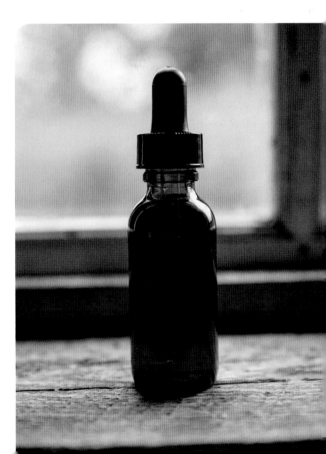

Vegetable glycerin is derived from fatty acid esters in coconut, soy, or palm oils. Vegetable glycerin extracts about one-third as well as alcohol, so if you use the same amount of plant material in vegetable glycerin as in alcohol, the medicine made with glycerin will be one-third as potent as the alcohol extraction.

NO NEED TO FREEZE

Some people suggest an additional step of putting the alcohol and the ground plant material in the freezer for 24 hours separately, combining them, and then putting the mixture back in the freezer to macerate. The reasoning is that less chlorophyll will be extracted. This is true, but it is not necessary or desirable for tincture making. This is a matter of aesthetics when making resin extract to smoke. People who make dabs (resin extract) are looking for a golden color, and they think chlorophyll lends an unpleasant taste. Another reason is that freezing reduces unwanted lipids and waxes in finished extract. But we want full-plant herbal medicine! Skip this step and use everything the cannabis plant has to offer.

HOW TO MAKE A TINCTURE

1. Decarboxylate if you want cannabinoids (rather than the acid form).

2. Grind flowers either by hand or in a blender.

3. Place ground flowers in a jar and add enough alcohol or glycerin to completely cover the plant material.

4. Let sit for 1 hour, shaking every 15 minutes. Or you can let it sit for 3 to 6 weeks and "shake and pray" as needed. If you want it to sit longer than an hour, pour into an appropriate-size mason jar with lid.

5. When the allotted time has passed, strain out the plant material.

6. Squeeze the plant material with your hands, cheesecloth, or an herb press to extract any remaining tincture, then compost the plant material.

7. Cover the tincture and let it sit overnight at room temperature.

8. The next day, strain the tincture through a pour-over coffee filter to remove all fine particulate matter left.

9. Transfer the tincture to small glass bottles with dropper tops. Label and store in a cool, dark place.

Pressing

For years, I simply used my hands to squeeze plant material and extract all I could from the plants. This works perfectly well for me because I grow my own plants and have lots of plant material to work with relatively inexpensively. But because working with cannabis can be time consuming and the plant material can be costly if purchased, it might serve you well to press the plant material more efficiently using a stainless-steel fruit wine press.

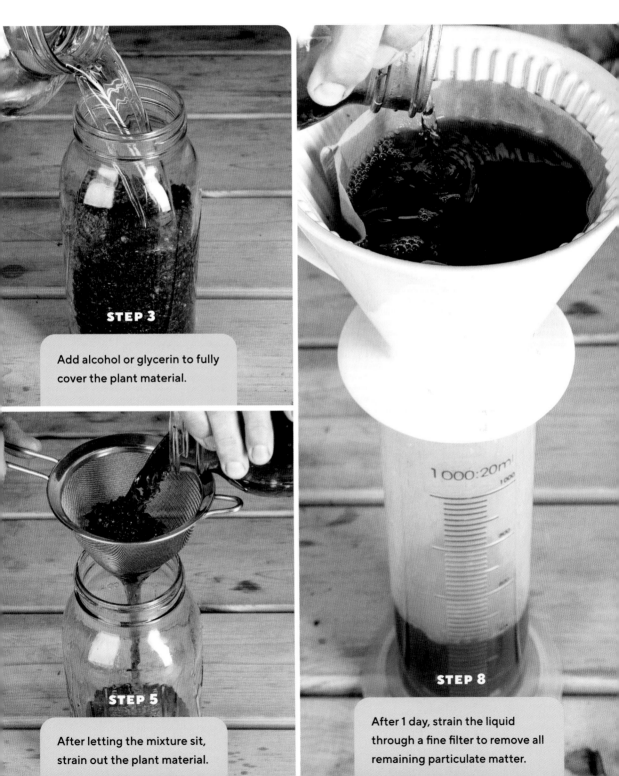

STEP 3

Add alcohol or glycerin to fully cover the plant material.

STEP 5

After letting the mixture sit, strain out the plant material.

STEP 8

After 1 day, strain the liquid through a fine filter to remove all remaining particulate matter.

Infused Oils

When plant material is placed in oil and heated, constituents will extract just like in a tincture. The difference is that extraction in oil needs heat to help pull the cannabinoids or acids into the oil solution. Saturated fats like coconut oil, fractionated coconut oil (MCT oil), butter, and ghee are excellent media for cannabis. The unsaturated fats in olive oil are also excellent solvents. Depending on which oil you choose, the cannabis medicine you make can be taken internally (the oil you use for these must be edible) or used topically.

Based on my lab-tested experience, the most potent oil infusions are done in a two-step process: First decarboxylate the plant material in the oven and then extract into the oil with heat. You have several options when it comes to the extraction step.

OVEN METHOD

Chop or grind your decarboxylated flowers into pea-size pieces and place them in an oven-safe pot. Cover the plant material with oil. Cover with a lid and place the pot in a 225°F (110°C) oven for at least 4 hours.

DOUBLE BOILER METHOD

Place pea-size decarboxylated flowers in a double boiler on the stovetop or wood stove and cover with oil. Cover the double boiler and heat over low heat for at least 4 hours, stirring occasionally.

SLOW-COOKER METHOD

Place pea-size decarboxylated flowers and oil in a slow cooker set on low (180°F/82°C) for at least 6 hours. Stir every hour.

BOTANICAL EXTRACTOR METHOD

If you're going to be making lots of infused oils, you may want to invest in a botanical extractor machine. Buy direct from the company to obtain the warranty (if you buy from an online retailer, you might lose the warranty option). The benefits of using this machine are that it heats and stirs automatically and it's easy to clean.

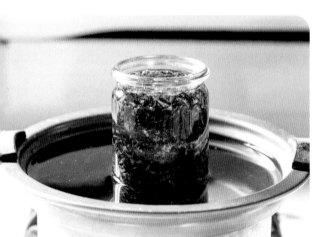

A double boiler is one good method for making infused oil.

Here's my tried-and-true method: Place decarboxylated plant material in a botanical extractor and cover with oil, following the volume guidelines provided with the machine. Set the temperature to 130°F (54°C), the lowest setting, and heat for 2 to 8 hours (I have not tested less than 8). Dance to the disco lights of the machine, come back in the allotted number of hours, and proceed with the final steps of making your oil.

FINISHING INFUSED OILS

Whatever extraction method you chose, at the end of the allotted time, strain the plant material from the oil, then press it with an herb press or squeeze in cheesecloth.

Compost the plant material and retain the oil. Let the infused oil sit overnight. Filter through cheesecloth (not a coffee filter) to remove fine particulate matter. Place in a cool, dry place; in the refrigerator; or in the freezer, depending on the storage requirements for the type of oil you used.

LABELING

Painter's tape is your friend. You can write on painter's tape with a marker and easily peel the tape off later and reuse the storage container. Label every single container you put your medicine in throughout the process of making it and storing it. Mark on the label: date, cultivar, solvent (oil or alcohol), and potency in mg/ml (if known).

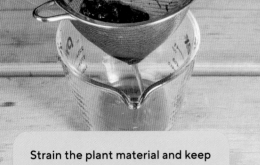

Strain the plant material and keep the oil. Let the oil sit overnight.

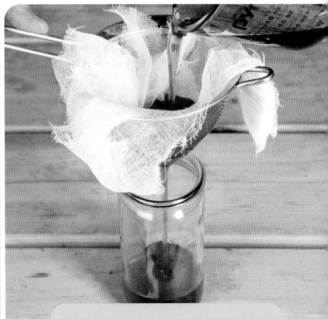

Filter the oil through a cheesecloth to remove any fine particulate matter.

Salves

The process of making salves is straight-forward. The simplest recipe is to take an infused oil, heat it with some beeswax, and, once the beeswax is melted, transfer the mixture to the container you want to dispense the salve from. Variations come in if you want different consistencies or to add additional ingredients like shea butter or coconut oil.

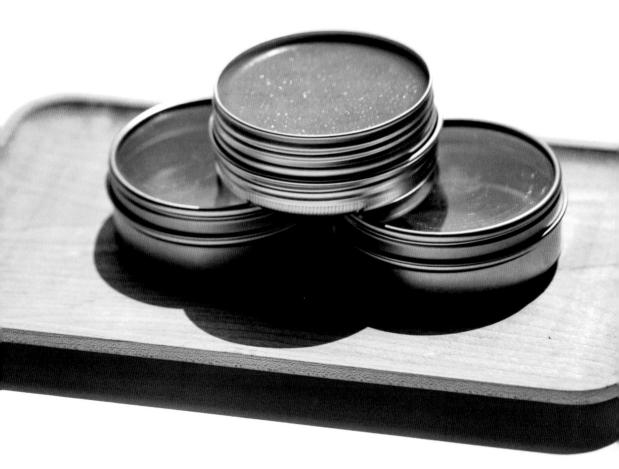

The Simplest Salve

Once you've made an infused oil with the plants that have the medicinal properties you want, you can strain it and make a salve. This is herbalist Rosemary Gladstar's tried-and-true salve recipe.

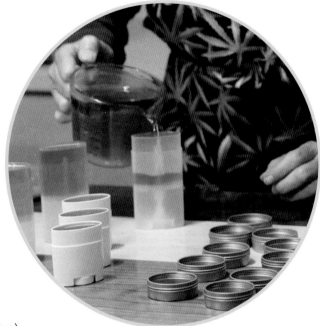

Ingredients

¾ cup infused herbal oil

¼ cup grated beeswax

1–2 tablespoons shea butter (optional as an added moisturizer)

1 tincture of benzoin or vitamin E capsule (optional as a preservative)

Instructions

1. Strain your infused oil.

2. For each ¾ cup oil, add ¼ cup beeswax. Grating the beeswax makes measuring and melting easier. Combine oil, beeswax, and shea butter (if using) in a double boiler and heat until the beeswax is completely melted. To check for consistency (density), place 1 tablespoon of the melted mixture in the freezer for just a minute or two. If it's too soft, add more beeswax; if too hard, add more oil.

3. Remove from the heat. Add the benzoin or vitamin E, if using (break open the capsule and pour it in). Immediately pour the salve into small glass jars or tins. Store any extra salve in a cool, dark place. Stored properly, salves will last for months, even years.

Note: Additional essential oils can be added right before pouring into containers.

Edibles

Once you have an infused oil of cannabis made with an oil safe for consumption like coconut oil or olive oil, you can take that infused oil and make it into something delicious. The only limits here are the limits of your creativity. Recipe books abound for cannabis edibles. Rather than focus on recipes, let's focus on some basic guidelines, especially for dosing.

If you are working strictly with CBD and not THC, there's no risk of the unexpected I-ate-too-much-of-an-edible-and-now-I-need-to-lie-down syndrome. The only "risk" with CBD is overconsuming when you don't need to. If we are using cannabis for health reasons and are wanting consistent dosing, the important thing is *knowing* what the dose is. For this reason, I recommend calculating dosage using the formula on page 102 or having your infused oil tested. If you only want to pay for one test, have the infused oil tested, then wait for the results before proceeding with the known milligrams of each cannabinoid you are working with.

HOW TO MAKE AN EDIBLE

1. Select a recipe that contains oil (or butter).

2. Make the infused oil you'll need.

3. Know the mg/ml of whatever cannabinoid you're working with (see Calculating Potency on page 113).

4. Convert mg/ml to teaspoons or tablespoons.
   5 ml = 1 teaspoon
   3 teaspoons = 1 tablespoon
   4 tablespoons = ¼ cup

5. Calculate the total mgs of cannabinoid in the whole batch.

6. Divide the total cannabinoids by the number of servings.

Cannabis Honey

Honey does not extract cannabinoids due to its hydrophilic (water-loving) nature. Cannabinoids are lipophilic (fat-loving). If you infuse cannabis flowers in honey, it will smell like cannabis, but you cannot draw out enough of the cannabinoids to make potent medicine. But don't disregard honey! It can be a nice addition to your medicine chest. You can powder cannabis flower and blend it into honey as a paste. In this case, you are not using honey to extract the cannabinoids; the honey becomes a delicious medium for the powdered cannabis flower.

Canna Energy Balls
(a.k.a. Tammi's Famous Goo Ballz)

This no-bake recipe is my favorite edible, using cannabis-infused coconut oil and combining some healthful ingredients like flaxseed, nut butter, and oats with a not-too-sweet finish from honey, vanilla, and chocolate chips. This will make 12 to 24 balls, depending on your dosage needs. If you want a stronger dose, make 12 balls. For a lighter dose, make 24.

Ingredients

- 1 tablespoon ground flaxseed
- 3 tablespoons hot water
- ¼ cup nut butter of choice (I like almond or peanut butter)
- 2–3 tablespoons honey or maple syrup
- 2 tablespoons cannabis-infused coconut oil
- ½ teaspoon vanilla extract
- ¼ teaspoon salt
- 1 cup oats (lightly toasted)
- ⅓ cup chopped walnuts
- ½ cup shredded coconut
- ⅓ cup chocolate chips

Instructions

1. Mix the flaxseed and hot water in a small bowl and let sit for 5 minutes.

2. Combine the flaxseed mixture, nut butter, honey, coconut oil, vanilla, and salt in a food processor.

3. Pulse in each of the following, one at a time: oats, walnuts, coconut, and chocolate chips.

4. Use a spoon to scoop out 12 to 24 portions.

5. Roll into balls and place on a cookie sheet.

6. Place in the refrigerator for at least 30 minutes.

These will store well in a sealed container for 2 weeks.

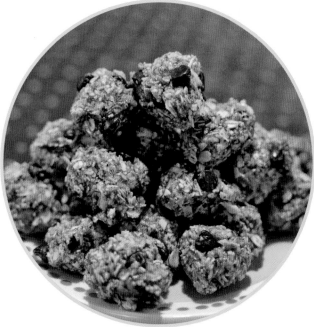

Testing

I like to have my flowers tested, make my medicine, calculate potency, and then have the tincture tested occasionally to see if I am extracting as well as I could be. Based on testing my own tinctures, I add a fudge factor of 10 percent when calculating potency. It's tough to decarboxylate and extract all the acid forms of constituents; some of the acid forms remain in the tincture, and some of the decarboxylated material remains in the plant material. We try for 100 percent, but it's usually closer to 90 percent of what the math says. I've bettered my fudge factor by weighing my plant material after I decarboxylate rather than before.

While testing and calculating your medicine's potency are good and informative steps and can help you understand how to use your home remedies, you can make beautiful medicine that helps people without testing or calculating. Our herbalist ancestors made amazing medicine without fancy lab equipment. You can develop a standardized process that delivers approximately the same potency in each batch of medicine you make.

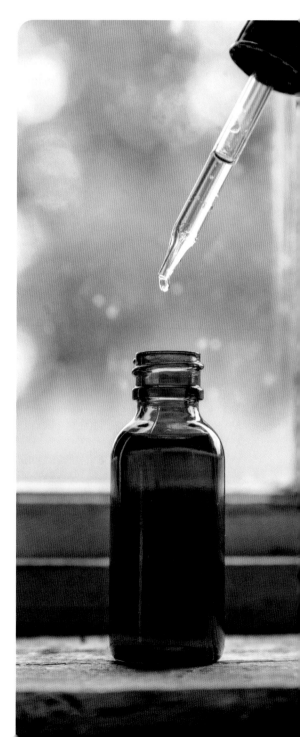

Calculating Potency

We can calculate the potency of our tincture, infused oil, or resin extract with some straightforward math. You must know three things: the potency of your flowers (from a lab test), the weight of the flowers in grams after you decarboxylate, and the volume in milliliters of infused oil or tincture at the end, after you've filtered out the plant material.

Here are a few standards of measurement. (Note that a "dropper" isn't necessarily full all the way up to the bulb. It's where the fluid naturally stops.)

DOING THE MATH

1. Weigh the plant material in grams after you have decarboxylated.

2. Convert to milligrams (multiply by 1,000).

3. Multiply percentage constituents from the lab test by milligrams of dried plant material (this tells you how many mg of CBD or THC you have in all the plant material you are using).

4. Make the medicine, strain, and measure the liquid in milliliters.

5. Divide milligrams of constituents by milliliters of liquid.

6. Multiply by a fudge factor of 90 percent.

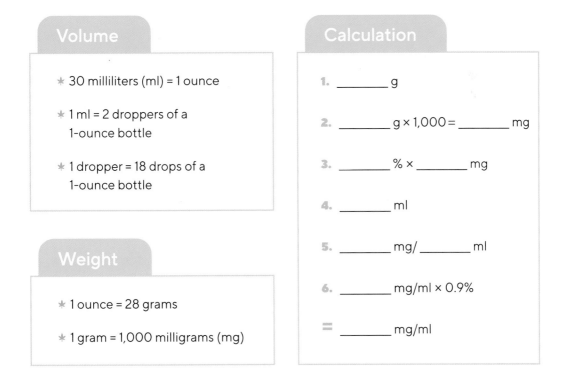

Volume

* 30 milliliters (ml) = 1 ounce

* 1 ml = 2 droppers of a 1-ounce bottle

* 1 dropper = 18 drops of a 1-ounce bottle

Weight

* 1 ounce = 28 grams

* 1 gram = 1,000 milligrams (mg)

Calculation

1. _____ g

2. _____ g × 1,000 = _____ mg

3. _____ % × _____ mg

4. _____ ml

5. _____ mg/ _____ ml

6. _____ mg/ml × 0.9%

= _____ mg/ml

Chapter 8

Using Cannabis Remedies

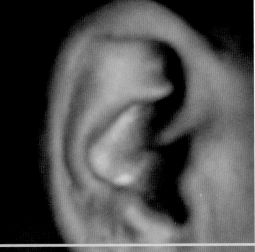

You've grown your cannabis, made your medicine, and have a basic understanding of what the different chemical constituents are useful for. Now it's time to take your medicine and learn what works.

How to Dose Appropriately

Cannabis is a low-dose botanical. It's not a plant to take medicinally in large quantities because a little bit can produce the desired effects we are looking for. High-THC cannabis can also induce an altered mental state. Work with the principle "Start low and go slow." Truly, start with a dose of one or two drops of a tincture, wait 2 hours, and see if you have the effects you are looking for. Starting with low doses is advisable because it allows you to pay close attention to what your body needs and to adjust accordingly. Too large a dose of THC could deter someone from taking the remedy in the future (not everyone likes to feel altered).

The effects of cannabis remedies taken orally (tinctures, edibles, oils) will last 5 to 8 hours, with a peak concentration at 4 to 6 hours on average. Dosing every 4 to 6 hours will keep cannabinoid levels constant, rather than rapidly fluctuating (as they do when inhaling smoke or vapor). The half-life of ingested cannabinoids is 18 to 32 hours. This means, for example, that 24 hours after a person ingests 10 mg of THC in an edible, she will still have approximately 5 mg of THC circulating in her blood.

The onset of effects after oral ingestion can take anywhere from 15 minutes (tinctures) to 3 hours (edibles), depending on stomach contents and liver function. This delay can be problematic for people who ingest cannabis orally and get impatient waiting for the effects (many people have a story about taking too many cannabis edibles because they don't feel the effects at first). A good rule of thumb is to wait at least 3 hours to see if effects occur. If, after 3 hours, effects are not felt, take one-fourth as much as the original dose and wait another 3 hours.

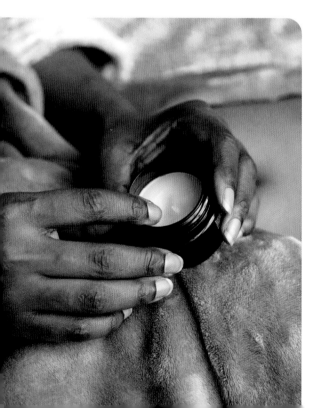

Minimum Effective Dose

What is the smallest dose that will produce a desired result? Start with 1 drop of tincture and wait 1 to 2 hours for effects to set in. If you don't feel the anticipated effects, take another dose. Wait. Once the optimum oral dose is found, take it, on average, every 4 to 6 hours to maintain blood levels.

I know the idea of minimum effective dose can be frustrating; some people want a specific measurement. However, people and plants are organic beings; no two are exactly alike. Get to know your body and the plant, then make educated decisions about the minimum effective dosage for your specific condition.

People new to cannabis as medicine will likely have a low tolerance and may feel effects at a very low dose of THC of 1 milligram or lower. Always start with a low dosage when starting a new round of medicine. Even people experienced with cannabis should start at a low dose with new formulas or a new version of a formula you've been working with.

THC to CBD Ratio

For most conditions, I recommend a 1:1 ratio of THC to CBD as the most potent and effective medicine. One benefit of this ratio is that CBD helps modulate some of the negative effects of THC, including anxiety and heart palpitations. Combining CBD with THC will also lengthen the desired effects of THC. Working together, CBD and THC have a potentiated effect, decreasing inflammation and pain more than either constituent alone. Balanced cannabinoids also lower the desire to use more. For people who are new to cannabis, I advise starting with cultivars higher in CBD before using cultivars higher in THC.

So, how do you know if you have a 1:1 ratio? The only way to determine this is to have your plants or finished medicine tested in a lab. You really can't know the potency of a specific cannabis plant unless you have it tested. Test results will give you the percentage of each of the cannabinoids within the flower.

The most straightforward way to get a 1:1 is to combine tinctures made from different plants, one high in THC and one high in CBD, for your final 1:1. Unless you find a plant with the 1:1 already inside it (they do exist but are not essential), you'll just need to do some math and careful measurements. Knowing how to do this enables you to get creative with your recipes. When you work with and understand one particular cultivar high in THC, you can pair it with high-CBD cultivars to make different formulations to address different conditions. That's when it gets fun!

Conditions

The most commonly reported conditions that people seek cannabis remedies for are anxiety, pain, and sleep problems. Cannabis remedies can be used for a wide range of conditions, and if you want more in-depth information on clinical applications, I go into detail in my previous book, *The Wholistic Healing Guide to Cannabis*. Here I will touch on dosage for common uses of home remedies.

Every person will react differently to a specific dosage and a particular cannabis cultivar. One cultivar might work well for a specific condition in one person and not in another. Therefore, we say "start low and go slow" in dosing so you can begin to understand if and how the particular medicine of cannabis is right for you.

ANXIETY

Given the nature of anxiety and the tendency for THC to cause anxiety, cultivar selection is crucial. High-CBD plants with very little THC are recommended to start. The terpene profile should also address specific anxiety symptoms. For example, if a person is anxious with low energy (depressed), stimulating terpenes like terpinolene and pinene are good choices, as are the uplifting floral (linalool) and citrus (limonene) terpenes. Higher myrcene levels will tend to be more sedating and grounding.

A good protocol is to start with 2.5 to 5.0 mg of high-CBD tincture every 6 to 8 hours. Increase the dosage to 50 mg if needed over a few weeks. When at an anxiolytic dose of CBD, THC can be added, starting with 1 mg of THC per dose. Remember the rule of minimum effective dose: More is not necessarily better. If you gain relief with 5 mg of CBD, there's no reason to use more.

PAIN

Pain-management doses start at a 1 mg oral dose of 1:1 THC:CBD every 4 to 6 hours, working up to 10 to 15 mg per dose if needed. Evidence suggests that increasing the dose above 15 mg does not increase pain relief.

SLEEP

Dose and delivery method are important in helping with sleep. In general, 1:1 extracts or high-THC extracts work better for sleep in the short term. For most people, CBD after 5:00 p.m. is too stimulating and should be avoided unless in a 1:1 ratio with THC. The dosing range is 1.5 to 15 mg of THC.

If you're having trouble falling asleep, take 1 or 2 drops of tincture 20 minutes before bed. If you're having trouble with waking up at night, you can try an edible 1 hour before bed. But remember to go low and slow with edibles, especially if you are new to cannabis. THC's psychoactive and intoxicating properties may interfere with restful sleep.

Contraindications

While cannabis is a safe and effective plant for home remedies, it also comes with a few contraindications for use and a few other considerations.

ADDICTION. Cannabis increases the amount of the neurotransmitter dopamine in the brain. Dopamine is the reward chemical that says, "Do that again!" This dopamine effect can lead to addiction for some people (cannabis has an addiction rate of 9 to 10 percent). However, while other addictive substances gradually cause a decrease in dopamine receptors, which creates a tolerance and the need for more of that substance to gain the same pleasurable effect, cannabis use does not decrease dopamine receptors. The risk for cannabis addiction increases if people begin using cannabis at a young age and use more potent forms. The quicker and more intensely a substance delivers a high, the higher the risk of addiction.

ALLERGIES. People can be allergic to cannabis, like any other plant. And people can develop allergies at any time in life. Windborne cannabis pollen can cause hay fever–like symptoms (this has been documented in the midwestern United States). Touching the plant can cause an allergic reaction on the skin for some people. Inhaling the vapor or smoke can cause respiratory allergies. Hempseed can also cause allergies in sensitive people.

ANXIETY. Relaxation and relief from anxiety are two of the most widely reported motives for working with cannabis. Cannabis is generally an effective treatment for anxiety, but there are a few situations where cannabis can cause anxiety. Cultivars with high THC, low CBD, and high levels of terpinolene terpenes, which tend to be stimulating, can contribute to anxiety. Some of these cultivars are bred for increased energy and alertness, and can result in zippy, anxious feelings. CBD mediates some of these negative effects of THC. I favor formulas with a more balanced THC-to-CBD ratio.

Too large a dose of THC can also cause anxiety. You cannot lethally overdose on cannabis the way you can with opioids, but too much THC can mimic the feeling of a panic attack.

One symptom of cannabis withdrawal is increased anxiety. If cessation of cannabis medicine is too abrupt, the body will not have enough time to restart production of endogenous cannabinoids and receptors. Ideally, users should taper use to zero over the course of 4 weeks to allow the body to increase production of its internal endocannabinoids.

Cannabis is not meant to take the place of psychotherapy, cognitive or behavioral therapy, or other emotional or psychological work. Cannabis is best used in a supportive role, due to her gift of fostering a sense of safety and well-being.

COGNITION. Cannabis use can cause some deficiency in attention, working memory, inhibition control, and decision-making ability when it is initially consumed. Long-term users can develop a tolerance to some of the negative effects of high-THC cultivars, such as acute memory deficiency, delayed reaction time, and decreased motor skills. People do not develop a tolerance to the desirable euphoric feeling.

In studying the long-term effects of cannabis use in adolescents, there is no evidence of a difference in IQ and achievement between users and nonusers. Cognitive deficiencies seen in adults disappear within 25 days of stopping cannabis use. There are, however, some concerns about the effects of cannabis on brain maturation in heavy cannabis users under age 25.

COMBINATION WITH OTHER DRUGS. Cannabis is an anti-inflammatory, anti-spasmodic, and anticonvulsant. It also modulates the immune system and reduces pain. If you are taking any other medications for similar relief, you should monitor the effects. Since cannabis does the same thing as these drugs, folks may find they can relieve their symptoms while decreasing the amount of the pharmaceutical being used, in consultation with their medical provider.

DEPLETION. In traditional Chinese medicine, cannabis is viewed as depleting to chi or vital energy. If you're planning to use cannabis long term, add a regimen of nourishing food and adaptogen herbs such as reishi mushroom, ashwagandha, or nettles to offset these depleting effects.

DEPRESSION. There is no evidence that cannabis users are more at risk of depression than anyone else. The "anti-motivational syndrome" of lethargy, apathy, and decreased productivity of cannabis users is a myth. No evidence exists for a causal relationship between cannabis and depression. There is evidence, however, that depressed individuals may be self-medicating with cannabis.

DETOXIFICATION PATHWAYS. Cannabis is eliminated from the body via the liver, through the same pathway as most pharmaceuticals. In a healthy liver, cannabis use alongside pharmaceuticals shouldn't be a problem. But as with all new regimens, assessment of the liver's detoxification function is important, so be aware of how your body is feeling. If you are on a pharmaceutical regimen, let your medical provider know you are using cannabis medicine.

DIARRHEA. High doses of THC (up to 1 gram per day) can cause diarrhea.

DROWSINESS. Drowsiness or sedation depends on dosage and cultivar. Both high doses of THC and CBD can cause sedation. Certain terpenes like myrcene can also be sedating.

DRY MOUTH AND RED EYES. A dry mouth and bloodshot eyes are symptoms of cannabis use in some people. If you have a tendency toward dryness, consider consuming moistening herbs such as marshmallow root in conjunction with cannabis.

HEART PROBLEMS. Initially, cannabis use may cause tachycardia (abnormally rapid heart rate) and hypotension (low blood pressure). People with a history of tachycardia or low blood pressure should consult with a physician before beginning a cannabis regimen. Long-term cannabis use can result in bradycardia (abnormally slow heart rate) and hypotension. The switch from tachycardia to bradycardia takes about 14 days of daily use of high-THC cannabis.

HYPOTENSION AND DIZZINESS. Cannabis use may cause hypotension (low blood pressure). When blood pressure drops, some people are prone to feeling dizzy when they stand up. After a few seconds, the body usually readjusts. This is more likely to occur with higher THC dosages.

IMMUNE FUNCTION. Animals that were given 50 to 100 times the psychoactive dose of cannabis showed a decrease in immunity. This is the equivalent of 1 gram for humans; most individuals working with cannabis for medicine will not regularly take a dose that high. No evidence exists that cannabis depletes the immune system when used at therapeutic levels. Normal immune systems have been seen in people with 20-year histories of regular cannabis use.

INSOMNIA. Cultivars that are high in THC and low in CBD can be too stimulating and cause sleeplessness (yes, low-dose CBD can be stimulating). A high-CBD cultivar doesn't necessarily promote sleep. It all depends on the terpene profile and the constituents of the particular cultivar.

NAUSEA. Nausea can be an unwanted effect of a high dose of THC. What is considered a "high dose" varies from person to person, but it is helpful to know this could happen. Animal studies have shown that CBD at low dosages decreases vomiting while higher doses of CBD increase it.

OVERDOSE. You cannot die from an overdose of cannabis, unlike opiates. Because the brain stem, the region of the brain that controls breathing and heart rate, lacks cannabinoid receptors, cannabis does not affect these essential bodily functions. If you've taken more than you planned or more than you feel comfortable consuming, sit in a quiet place and rest until the body can metabolize the THC. Calamus root or Ghost Pipe tincture can help.

PARANOIA. One of the gifts of cannabis is to help us open, neurochemically, into a sense of safety. But some people who use cannabis when they are in a vulnerable time or place might feel resistance, which can manifest in a sense of paranoia. It is advisable, especially for new cannabis users, to begin with low doses in secure, comforting surroundings.

PREGNANCY. While there is documented evidence of women using cannabis to mitigate pain associated with menstrual and reproductive issues, including migraines, cramps, and leg pain, it is not advisable to use cannabis during pregnancy without supervision of your obstetrician or midwife. Because the endocannabinoid system is involved in fetal neural development, abstaining from cannabis use during pregnancy is advised. When a pregnant woman consumes cannabis, THC and CBD do cross the placenta and reach the fetus (albeit at a low level, 0.8 percent of mom's blood level). Limited use of cannabis for morning sickness or pain management should be weighed against potential risks.

PSYCHOSIS. Over the last several decades, cannabis use has increased in the general population while the incidence of psychosis has remained the same. Individuals who are predisposed to psychosis should avoid cultivars that are high in THC due to its psychomimetic properties.

RESPIRATORY ISSUES. Studies show no decrease in lung function or increased risk of lung cancer in 20-year cannabis-only smokers. When cannabis is combined with tobacco, all the risk factors for tobacco appear because of tobacco. Long-term cannabis smokers have a modestly increased risk of bronchitis, but upon cessation or use of a vaporizer the risk diminishes.

TOLERANCE. People develop tolerance to cannabis. To achieve the same effects over time, higher doses need to be consumed. When taking the minimum effective dose, tolerance can develop in as little as 2 weeks, which may require increasing the dose to get the desired effect.

WITHDRAWAL. If you are taking a cannabis remedy for a period of time and then suddenly stop taking it, your body will need time to readjust, and you may feel withdrawal symptoms while it does. It takes about 3 weeks for your endocannabinoid system to rebalance. Withdrawal from cannabis might be uncomfortable, but it's never lethal. Withdrawal symptoms from cannabis begin 1 to 2 days after cessation of use and include irritability, anxiety, decreased appetite, restlessness, sleep disturbance, and sometimes functional impairment. Symptoms usually peak at 1 week and persist for 3 to 4 weeks. After 4 weeks, your cannabinoid receptors return to normal and symptoms disappear. It's important to note that if people have been working with cannabis to treat anxiety, going through withdrawal might trigger a surge of anxiety, and those people may feel the need to start using cannabis again; they will need to ride out the withdrawal symptom of anxiety to reach equilibrium.

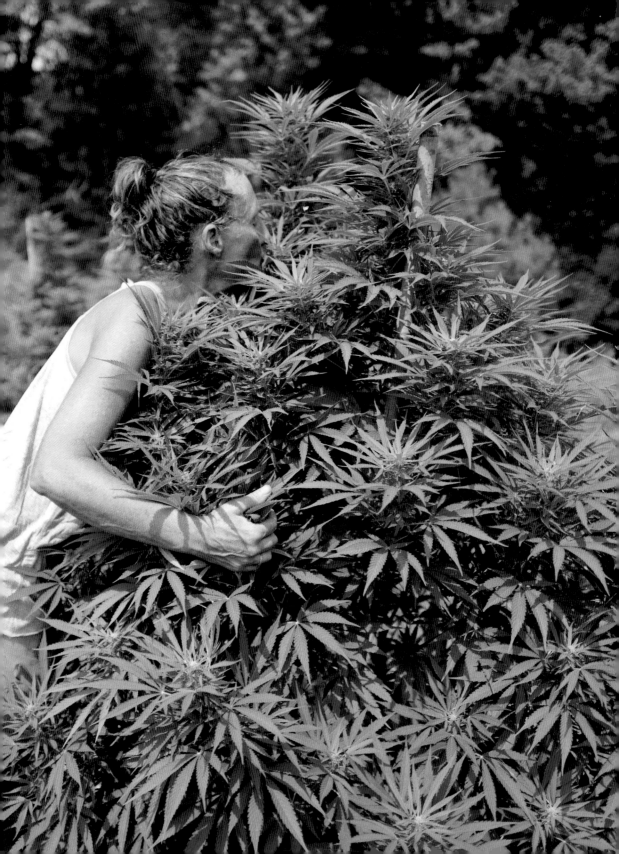

Appendix

Sourcing Cannabis for Medicine

What if you are not going to grow cannabis yourself? Can you buy cannabis and still make good medicine? Yes.

Cannabis is a plant. Source it like you would any other plant you would use to create therapeutic remedies. It's best to use local, organic, and pesticide-free plants. It's important to know the conditions the plant was grown in. The best way to ensure the quality of your cannabis is to get to know a grower, build a relationship, and ask questions.

Build a Relationship with a Grower

One of the most important aspects of good medicine is a good relationship with where it comes from. It's not just about getting a good deal today, it's an investment in a long-term connection to where your medicine is coming from.

Early in the growing season (in spring), have a conversation with local growers about purchasing flowers at the end of the season. Most states in which cannabis cultivation is legal provide a list of licensed growers on the state's agricultural website.

Find a grower who has a deep respect and love for their plants. Your medicine begins with the relationship of the human interacting with your flowers and the environment the flowers grow in. My advice is not to grill the grower with questions, but I do want to offer you a sense of the kinds of things you want to know about how your medicine is made.

The following is helpful for buying both "hemp" and high-THC cannabis for medicine making and it's written primarily for buying hemp. When buying high-THC cannabis, you don't need smokable grade (this is the most expensive), but you could ask all the same questions and purchase the trimmed sugar leaves from the trimming process.

Questions for the Grower

HOW IS THE PLANT GROWN?

Ask about their approach to growing. Cannabis, like any crop, can be grown using a large-scale agricultural model or a smaller-scale horticultural model. Large-scale "throw-and-grow" farmers plant hemp like industrial corn. They crowd as many plants as possible into a plot and use petroleum-based fertilizers that ultimately deplete the soil and the life around the fields. This model lacks perspective on what we will leave for the next generation and how much we can take from the land and soil without depleting it. Every harvest removes biomass and nutrients from the land.

We must help farmers transition away from this depleting model into a more sustainable and regenerative one. A more holistic model starts from the belief that we are part of, and interconnected with, the world around us, and we must work to improve our natural environment, starting with the soil. Biodynamic, permaculture, and regenerative growing philosophies all utilize this perspective in their growing practices. My growing philosophy centers around healthy soil.

HOW MANY PLANTS DO YOU GROW?

The number of plants will give you an idea of how much time they could potentially be spending with the plants. Someone managing 10 acres of 1,500 plants per acre has a different relationship with them than someone managing a total of 200 plants. This question helps you understand how much time and care the grower can offer their plants.

WHAT ARE YOU GROWING FOR?

You want the grower to be growing for "smokable grade flowers." It's about the quality of the plant grown. "Smokable grade" means high quality. Even if you don't intend to use the flowers for smoking, the "smokable" nomenclature is about top quality. The farmer who is growing smokable grade flowers will spend more time harvesting, drying, trimming, and curing the flowers. These farmers are growing different cultivars with quality in mind. The smokable market brings the top dollar to the grower and requires more skill and knowledge to produce the highest grade of flower. These flowers will look green or purple, not brown. There should be zero stems and zero bigger fan leaves covering the dried flower. The flower should be trimmed down and should have few smaller leaves visible over the flower.

Many big farms grow "hemp" for biomass. You want to steer away from these farms. The plants are packed in together, with little or no time for individual inspection or care. It's all about the numbers. These plants will be quickly heat-dried and ground up for processing. Even if the farmer is only processing flowers rather than the whole plant, they are usually drying the flowers with heat on conveyors. This process evaporates all the terpenes, which are the molecules you want in your medicine.

HOW DO YOU MANAGE PESTS? WHAT ARE YOUR PRACTICES DURING THE FLOWERING PHASE?

Regulations vary from state to state, and organic practices aren't enough with regard to a flower you might smoke or concentrate. What you really want to know is, what are they spraying on the plants during flowering? Ideally the answer is "nothing." Large farms with thousands of plants won't spray anything because they've got the numbers. Sometimes inexperienced farmers believe if it's "organic" it's okay to spray on the flowers. This is not usually correct. Very few interventions are safe and acceptable. Look to California policy for what they consider safe to be sprayed on cannabis flowers.

HAVE YOU TESTED YOUR FLOWERS?

Do they have a Certificate of Analysis (COA)? All legal growers must test for THC levels to be compliant for "hemp" and present the results in the form of a COA to their state. The benefit to you is you can get these test results for the flowers you are buying, which will be helpful when you make medicine and want to calculate its potency. Terpene test results are an added bonus but are not the norm.

WHAT IS YOUR ASKING PRICE FOR FLOWERS?

Do they offer a lower rate if you buy in bulk? Prices vary wildly in the hemp market, even in the smokable flower market. Don't bother buying smaller than ¼ pound (114 grams) for making medicine; ¼ pound will make roughly a quart of tincture or infused oil.

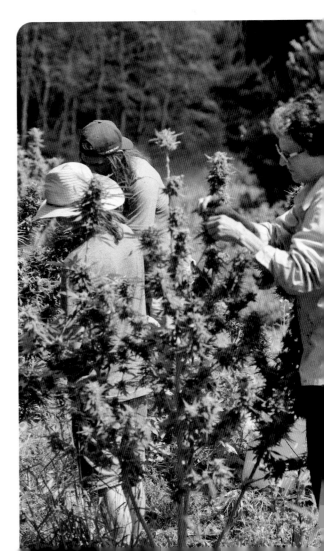

How to Help Your Grower

Offer to prepurchase the flowers. This is the CSA (community-supported agriculture) model. You don't need the grower to have a formal CSA program, you can simply negotiate and reserve the quantity of flowers you will need in advance.

Offer to help with the harvest. Like many harvests, cannabis demands a tremendous amount of work in a short amount of time. There is always room for another helping hand for trimming and processing flowers.

Cook a nice meal. Whether it's for the grower or for them to share with their crew, a nice meal is a heartfelt gesture of friendship, and it's incredibly helpful during the busy harvest time.

Buying CBD Products

What if you're not growing cannabis or making medicine, but you still want to use cannabis medicinally? When you, as a consumer, walk into a store to buy a high-CBD cannabis product, you are entering a wild and unregulated arena. You can't be sure that what the manufacturer says is in the product is actually in there or at the concentrations they report. Currently, no regulations or accountability exist for the labels "full-spectrum" or "whole-plant extract" on CBD products. The question for many consumers is, "Where do I get quality medicine?" If you don't have the time or desire to make your own, try to buy from a local herbalist who makes tinctures or infused oils and knows plant medicine. If you are buying from a cannabis dispensary, there are some things to educate yourself about.

You want your medicine to contain everything the plant made while it was growing: cannabinoids, terpenes, flavonoids, fats, waxes, and chlorophyll. Some commercial extractors will remove one or more of these. You want these things from the plant itself, not added in from another source. Terpenes are sometimes added in from another plant. Ask your dispensary salesperson the following questions.

IS THIS MADE FROM ORGANIC FLOWERS? You want organic flowers.

HOW ARE THEY EXTRACTING? If the answer is "with butane," move on. Ethanol or supercritical carbon dioxide are the industry standards. Home medicine makers usually use ethanol or butane, but I advise against using butane.

DO THEY TEST THE END PRODUCT FOR HEAVY METALS, PESTICIDES, AND MOLD?

You want medicine free from heavy metals, pesticides, and mold. Ask to see the test results. You are paying top dollar, and this is one of the benefits of it.

WHEN THEY EXTRACT, WHAT ARE THEY TAKING OUT AND WHAT ARE THEY LEAVING IN?

Sometimes the flowers come in a little "hot," containing more than the legal 0.3 percent THC. Some companies remove enough THC to bring the level below the legal limit. You want the legal limit of THC. If they take anything else out, you don't want the product.

DOES IT SMELL LIKE CANNABIS?

You should be able to smell the terpenes. If it doesn't smell like cannabis, it's made with isolate, doesn't have terpenes, and you don't want it. Your edibles should taste and smell like weed.

AFTER THEY'VE EXTRACTED, ARE THEY PUTTING ANYTHING ELSE BACK IN?

If they have, you don't want the product. Companies often use additives to compensate for poor-quality starting flowers, most commonly CBD isolate.

IS THERE ANY ISOLATE IN THE PRODUCT?

If the answer is yes, you don't want it. Some companies will use full-plant extraction and then add isolated CBD or THC back into the product.

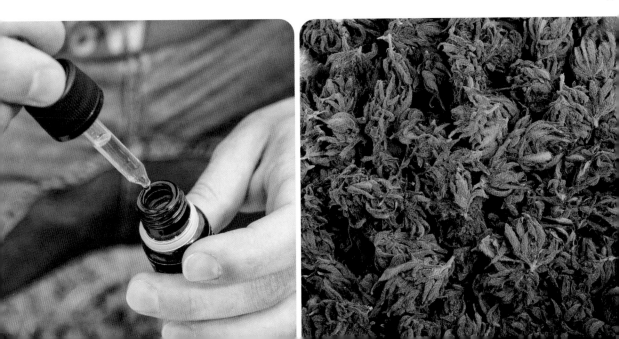

Resources

Seed companies

OREGON CBD has set the standard for high-CBD genetics. I use their seeds and trust them for my students to grow successfully as well.
http://oregoncbdseeds.com

COLORADO CBD SEED offers unique high-CBD cultivars. I love the purple Abacus cultivar, and this breeder works with Abacus as the parent stock.
https://coloradocbdseed.com

ORGANIGROW CANADA is run by Alexis Burnett, who has been breeding and growing for many years in the Northeast. He is known for high-THC cultivars but also has some high-CBD cultivars in the mix as well.
https://organigrowcanada.com

HUMBOLDT SEED COMPANY has been breeding for years and has an awesome reputation. You cannot purchase directly from them, but you can research distributors on their website and find places to purchase seeds.
https://humboldtseedcompany.com

GOAT AND MONKEY SEEDS is based in Massachusetts and is a quality breeder in the Northeast.
https://goatandmonkey.com

REGENERATIVE SEED COMPANY is based in Oregon and has been cultivating, breeding, and growing outdoors for many years.
https://regenerativeseeds.com

Tools for growing

FELCO makes my favorite clippers and hand pruners.
https://felco.com

ARBICO ORGANICS offers a wide variety of organic gardening supplies and natural pest control solutions.
https://arbico-organics.com

Insect control

Beneficial Insectary
https://insectary.com

Biobest
https://biobestgroup.com

Biobee
https://biobee.com

Lab testing

Nelson Analytical Lab
www.nelsonanalytical.com

Soil

Rabbit Creek Farm
https://easygrowsoil.com

Further Reading

The Cannabis Grow Bible:
The Definitive Guide to Growing Marijuana for Recreational and Medical Use (3rd edition) by Greg Green (Green Candy Press, 2017)

Ed Rosenthal's Marijuana Grower's Handbook:
Your Complete Guide for Medical and Personal Marijuana Cultivation by Ed Rosenthal (Quick American, 2009)

Feminist Weed Farmer:
Growing Mindful Medicine in Your Own Backyard by Madrone Stewart (Microcosm, 2018)

Handbook of Cannabis
edited by Roger G. Pertwee (Oxford University Press, 2014)

Handbook of Cannabis for Clinicians:
Principles and Practice by Dustin Sulak, DO (W. W. Norton & Company, 2021)

Hemp Diseases and Pests:
Management and Biological Control by J. M. McPartland, R. C. Clarke, and D. P. Watson (CABI, 2000)

Homegrown Cannabis:
A Beginner's Guide to Cultivating Organic Cannabis (Volume 3) by Alexis Burnett (Union Square & Co., 2021)

Marijuana Garden Saver:
Handbook for Healthy Plants by J. C. Stitch, edited by Ed Rosenthal (Quick American, 2008)

Marijuana Horticulture:
The Indoor/Outdoor Medical Grower's Bible by Jorge Cervantes (Van Patten, 2006)

Marijuana Horticulture Fundamentals:
A Comprehensive Guide to Cannabis Cultivation and Hashish Production by K of Trichome Technologies and Kenneth Morrow (Green Candy Press, 2016)

Marijuana Pest and Disease Control:
How to Protect Your Plants and Win Back Your Garden by Ed Rosenthal with Kathy Imbriani (Quick American, 2012)

Mycorrhizal Planet:
How Symbiotic Fungi Work with Roots to Support Plant Health and Build Soil Fertility by Michael Phillips (Chelsea Green, 2017)

The Wholistic Healing Guide to Cannabis:
Understanding the Endocannabinoid System, Addressing Specific Ailments and Conditions, and Making Cannabis-Based Remedies by Tammi Sweet (Storey, 2020)

Metric Conversions

Unless you have finely calibrated measuring equipment, conversions between US and metric measurements will be somewhat inexact. It's important to convert the measurements for all of the ingredients in a recipe to maintain the same proportions as the original.

Weight

To convert	to	multiply
ounces	grams	ounces by 28.35
pounds	grams	pounds by 453.5
pounds	kilograms	pounds by 0.45

US	Metric
0.035 ounce	1 gram
¼ ounce	7 grams
½ ounce	14 grams
1 ounce	28 grams
1¼ ounces	35 grams
1½ ounces	40 grams
1¾ ounces	50 grams
2½ ounces	70 grams
3½ ounces	100 grams
4 ounces	113 grams
5 ounces	140 grams
8 ounces	228 grams
8¾ ounces	250 grams
10 ounces	280 grams
15 ounces	425 grams
16 ounces (1 pound)	454 grams

Volume

To convert	to	multiply
teaspoons	milliliters	teaspoons by 4.93
tablespoons	milliliters	tablespoons by 14.79
fluid ounces	milliliters	fluid ounces by 29.57
cups	milliliters	cups by 236.59
cups	liters	cups by 0.24
pints	milliliters	pints by 473.18
pints	liters	pints by 0.473
quarts	milliliters	quarts by 946.36
quarts	liters	quarts by 0.946
gallons	liters	gallons by 3.785

US	Metric
1 teaspoon	5 milliliters
1 tablespoon	15 milliliters
¼ cup	60 milliliters
½ cup	120 milliliters
1 cup	240 milliliters
1¼ cups	300 milliliters
1½ cups	355 milliliters
2 cups	480 milliliters
2½ cups	600 milliliters
3 cups	710 milliliters
4 cups (1 quart)	0.95 liter
4 quarts (1 gallon)	3.8 liters

About the Author

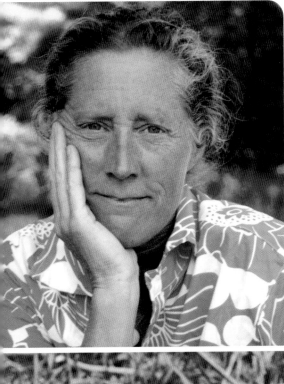

Tammi Sweet is a practitioner and teacher of herbal medicine. She is deeply influenced by her studies with herbalists Rosemary Gladstar, Pam Montgomery, Brooke Medicine Eagle, Tom Brown, Jr., and by Stephen Buhner's pioneering work on the heart as an organ of perception. Sweet has taught herbalism and physiology in colleges, massage schools, and herbal clinics throughout the United States. In 2007, she set out to combine her areas of interest into one curriculum and to teach them in ways that made sense to her. So, she cofounded the Heartstone Center for Earth Essentials near Ithaca, New York, with her partner, Kris Miller, where they offer herbalist programs, an herbal apprenticeship, and a Journey of the Heart course. They also offer online courses that integrate physiology and plant medicine. Sweet's mission for Heartstone is to co-create, with the land, a space where people can come home, take refuge, find the sacred, and facilitate healing.

Go behind the scenes in Tammi Sweet's kitchen, garden, and classroom. Access her free online video series on growing cannabis, making medicine, and the endocannabinoid system at:
www.heart-stone.com/cannabis

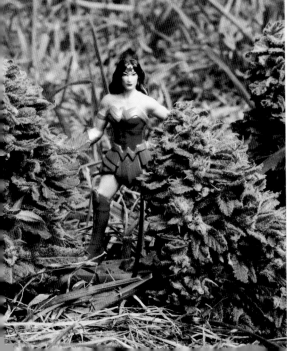

Index

Page numbers in *italics* indicate photos; numbers in **bold** indicate charts.

Heal Yourself Naturally
with More Books from Storey

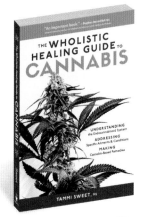

The Wholistic Healing Guide to Cannabis by Tammi Sweet, MS

This guide provides a deep understanding of the science behind cannabis medicine, including the chemistry of the cannabis plant, the physiology of the body's endocannabinoid system, and preparation and dosage guidelines for addressing a wide range of ailments, including stress, anxiety, chronic pain, insomnia, and more.

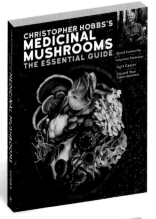

Christopher Hobbs's Medicinal Mushrooms: The Essential Guide

Hobbs introduces you to the mushroom varieties most widely used for health and healing, discussing their powerful benefits and the science behind their effectiveness, and shows you how to make mushroom medicine at home.

Rosemary Gladstar's Medicinal Herbs: A Beginner's Guide

Craft a soothing aloe lotion for poison ivy or make a dandelion-burdock tincture to aid sluggish digestion! Gladstar profiles 33 common healing plants and shows you how to grow, harvest, prepare, and use them in healing tinctures, oils, and creams.

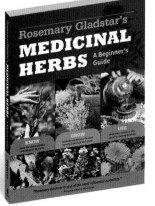

Join the conversation. Share your experience with this book, learn more about Storey Publishing's authors, and read original essays and book excerpts at storey.com. Look for our books wherever quality books are sold or call 800-441-5700.